Balanced
B O O B S

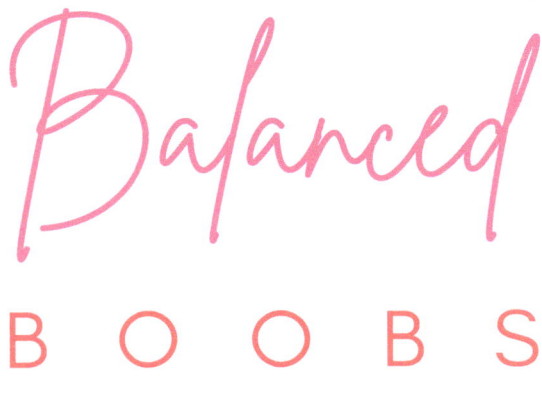

Harnessing the Power of Lymphatic Breast Health. is a practical guide that helps you unlock the secrets of your body's lymphatic system, empowering you to achieve balance and optimal breast health.

BY SUMMER L. MAIDEN LMT, NMT

Balanced Boobs: Harnessing the Power of Lymphatic Breast Health

Copywrite © 2024 by Summer L. Maiden, LMT, NMT

All rights reserved. No part of this publication may be reproduced, distributed, or transmitted in any form or by any means, including photocopying, recording, or other electronic or mechanical methods, without the prior written permission of the publisher, except in the case of brief quotations embodied in critical reviews and specific other noncommercial uses permitted by copyright law.

For permission requests, contact the author/self-publisher at:
Summer Maiden, LMT, NMT
Email/www.waze2wellness.com

Book and Cover design by Summer Maiden, LMT, NMT

Disclaimer: This book is intended for informational purposes only. It is not a substitute for professional medical advice, diagnosis, or treatment. Always seek the advice of your physician or qualified health provider with any questions you may have regarding a medical condition.

ISBN: 979-8-9917720-3-7

First Edition 2024

Printed in the United States of America

Dedication

This book is dedicated to the losses and survivorship of family and loved ones who have bravely endured the battle against breast cancer.

In loving memory of Aunt Roberta Johnson, whose spirit and strength will never be forgotten.

To my mentor, Susan Edgar, a two-time survivor whose courage continues to inspire me every day.

To my dear friend Janene John, also a two-time survivor whose resilience has been a beacon of hope.

And to my cousin Lisa Maiden, a survivor whose determination is a testament to the power of perseverance.

You all are the heart of this dedication, and your strength lives on to encourage others to promote breast health through these pages.

TABLE OF CONTENTS

Welcome to Balanced Boobs

1	Anatomy of the Breast	15
2	Benefits of Breast Health	20
3	The Lymphatic Role in Breast Health	55
4	Holistic Approach to Breast Health	63
5	Lymphatic Massage Techniques	71
6	Diet and Lifestyle for Health Breast	81

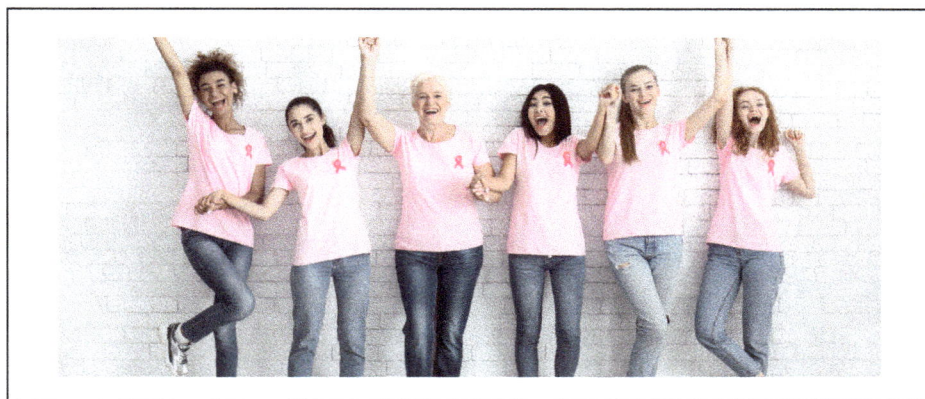

Welcome to Balanced Boobs!

Breast lymphatic health plays a vital role in women's overall wellness. By comprehending the intricate anatomy and recognizing the significance of safeguarding breast health, women can become proactive in their breast care. The lymphatic system, often neglected, is essential for detoxification, fluid regulation, and breast tissue support.

This book explores the critical elements of breast lymphatic health, equipping you with the essential knowledge to make informed choices about your breast health. With a deeper understanding of this system, you will readily identify any structural variations or irregularities that may occur.

Furthermore, we will explore prevalent breast health concerns and emphasize the critical need for early detection and timely intervention.

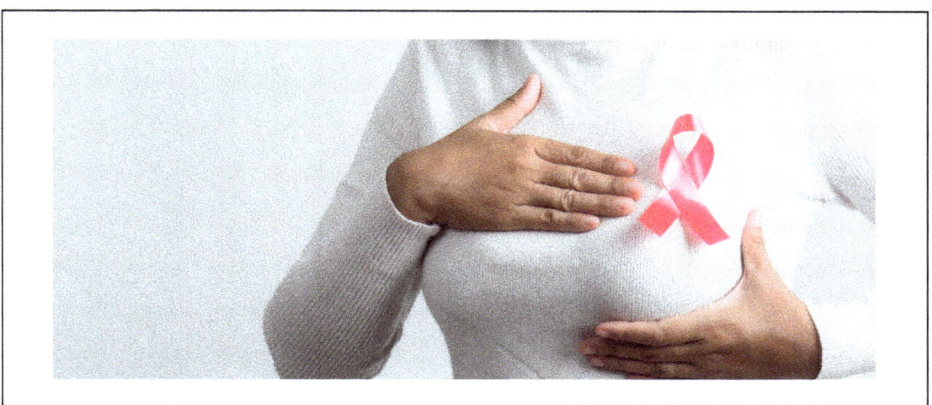

ACKNOWLEDGEMENTS

Writing a book is never a solitary journey, and my heart is filled with gratitude for the many people who have walked beside me and offered their support, making this endeavor possible.

First and foremost, I am deeply thankful to God for the wisdom and strength that have guided me through this process. To my family and closest friends, your unwavering love and belief in me have been my most significant source of encouragement. Your support has carried me through every challenge; I am forever grateful.

I also want to extend my heartfelt empathy and gratefulness to the women in my life who have passed and survived this breast health journey.

This book reflects the love, faith, and support I've received as much as it does the work that went into it. Thank you all.

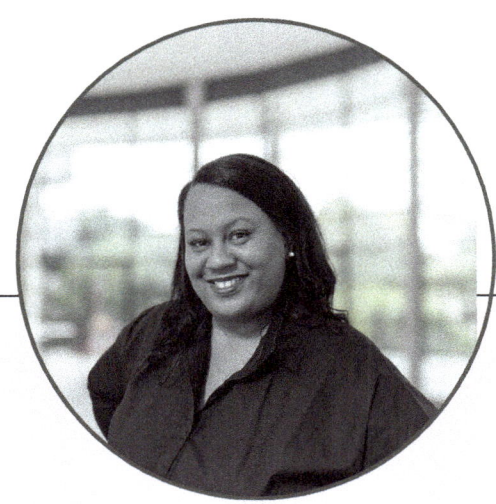

About the author

As a Licensed Massage Therapist with over eighteen years of experience, I specialize in Manual Lymphatic Drainage Massage. My certifications in Breast Health enable me to guide women in maintaining healthy breast practices and provide support before and during post-surgical recovery following breast surgeries.

Having witnessed both the losses and survivorship associated with Breast Cancer among my loved ones, I am deeply committed to educating others about alternative therapies that promote pain relief, enhance immunity, foster self-care, and support lymphatic health. I have applied this therapeutic approach across various fields, including General Health, Hematology/Oncology, Cardiac, Pulmonary, Post-Surgery, Pregnancy, and Rehabilitation.

Summer Maiden

Chapter 1
Anatomy of the Breast

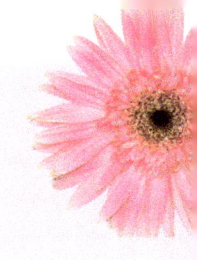

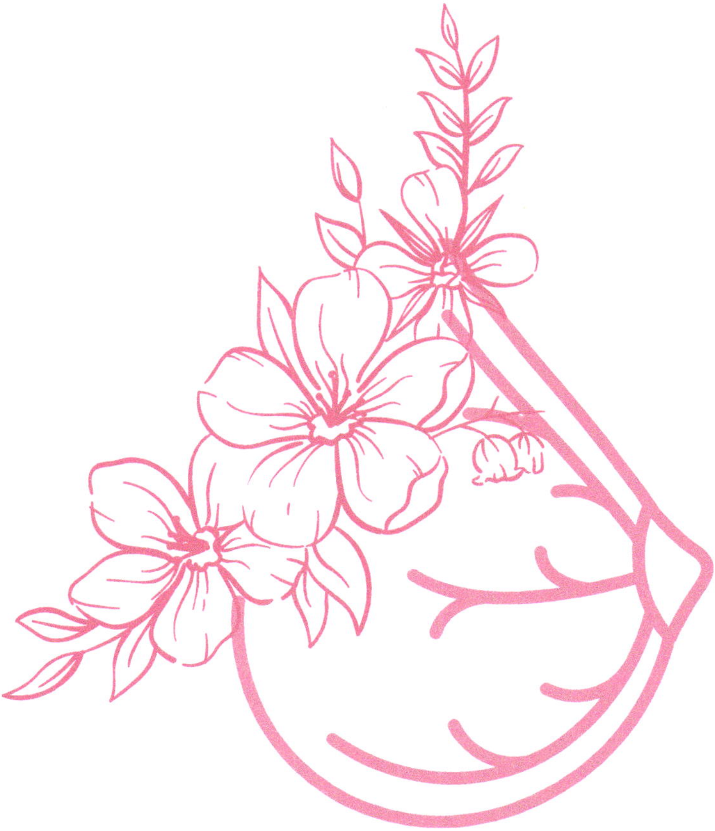

Anatomy of the Breast

Best health practices facilitate Good Breast Health; it is helpful to begin by learning about the anatomy of the breast so you can better understand how to care for and monitor your breast health. Tissues, lobes, glands, and ducts form women's breasts. Some lobes contain milk-producing glands called lobules, which connect to ducts that carry milk to the nipple.

Understanding the essential parts can assist you in effectively monitoring your breast health. For example, knowing the location of the lobes and ducts within the breast can help you recognize any unusual changes should they occur.

Glandular Tissue:
- The tissue responsible for producing milk during lactation is called Glandular Tissue. This Gladular Tissue consists of lobes and lobules, where milk production happens, and ducts carrying the milk to the nipple.

Ducts:
- Ducts are small tubes that transport milk from the lobules to the nipple. During breastfeeding, milk is released through the terminal ducts at the end of the nipples.

Anatomy of the Breast

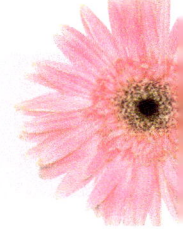

Fatty Tissue:
- The breast contains fatty tissue, which surrounds and cushions the glandular tissue and ducts. The amount of breast adipose (fat) tissue varies among individuals and contributes to its size and shape. Weight gain can also contribute to this fatty tissue.

Connective Tissue:
- The connective tissue in the breast provides structural support. Ligaments maintain the shape and position of the breast.

Blood Vessels:
- Blood vessels supply oxygen and nutrients to breast tissue, and they play an imperative role in maintaining its health and functionality.

Lymphatic Vessels:
- The lymphatic system is an essential part of the immune system. It helps to remove waste, toxins, and excess fluid from breast tissue. Lymphatic vessels transport lymph fluid to lymph nodes, which filter out harmful substances.

Anatomy of the Breast

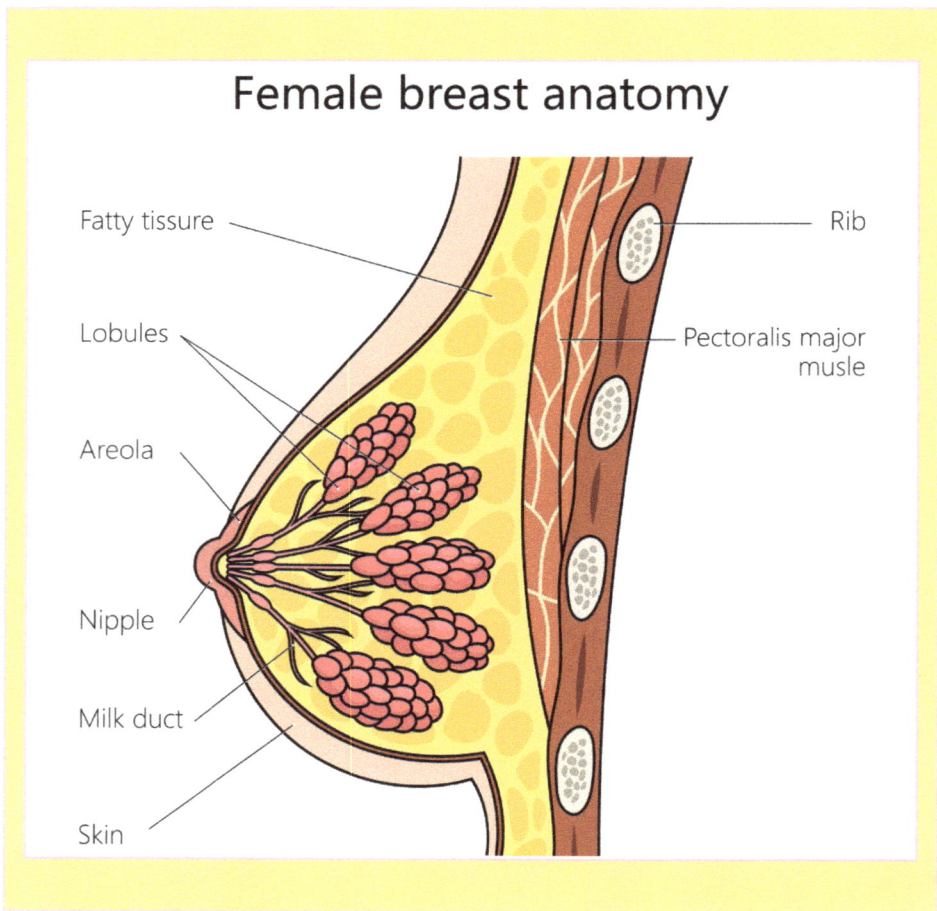

Anatomy of the Breast

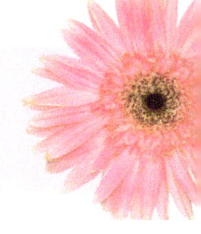

Being aware of the anatomy and regular self-examination of the standard look and feel of your breasts can help you detect any unusual changes early. Prioritizing your breast health is a significant step toward overall wellness and peace of mind.

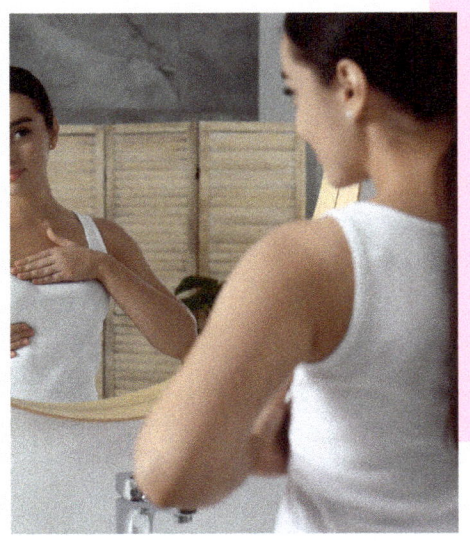

"Performing self-examinations regularly and being aware of the normal look and feel of your breasts can help you detect any unusual changes early."

Chapter 2
Benefits of Breast Health

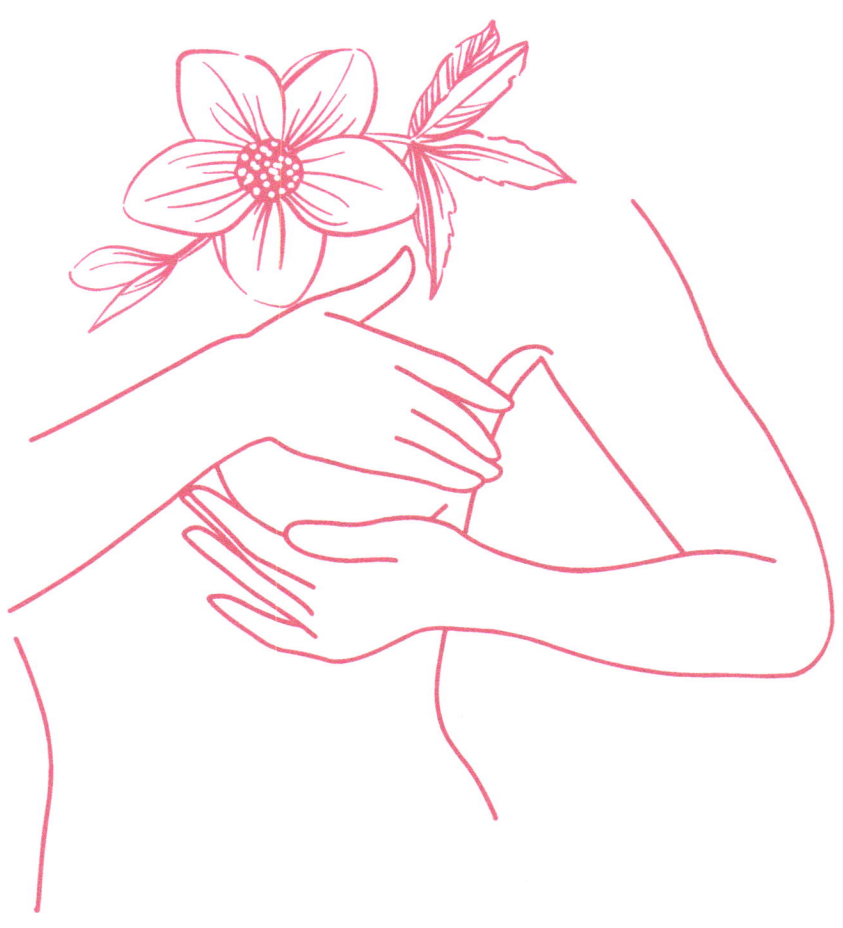

Benefits of Breast Health

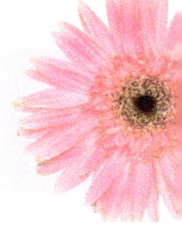

Maintaining good breast health is vital for detecting diseases early, such as breast cancer. Regular self-examinations, clinical exams, mammograms, and thermography are essential practices. It is crucial to maintain good breast health to detect diseases such as breast cancer early. Risk factors, healthy lifestyle choices, staying informed, and awareness of potential issues are involved in understanding breast health. Here are a few considered essential practices:

- **Self-Examinations:**

Regular self-examination is crucial for maintaining breast health. It is recommended that you keep a journal for monthly check-ins or when you notice any changes in the size, shape, or color of your breasts. Self-exams help you identify any changes that may not be immediately apparent. You should also feel your breasts for lumps or textures (the entire protocol is provided later in the self-care section). Becoming familiar with the everyday look and feel of your breasts makes it easier to notice any changes.

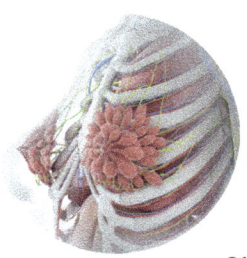

Benefits of Breast Health

Clinical Breast Exam (CBE)
A clinical breast exam is a physical examination of the breasts performed by a healthcare professional, such as a doctor, nurse, or breast health specialist, to check for lumps, changes in breast size or shape, skin changes, or any abnormalities in the breasts and underarm areas. The provider will use their hands to feel for any unusual masses or thickening in the breast tissue.

The healthcare professional manually examines the breasts and underarms for lumps or abnormalities. This is typically done during routine annual checkups, especially for women aged 20 and older. It is non-invasive, requires no special equipment, and can detect physical changes. Because smaller lumps or abnormalities may be missed and undetectable by touch alone in an office setting, this is why self-exams are also essential.

Mammograms:
A mammogram is a specialized X-ray imaging technique used to examine breast tissue for early signs of breast cancer, such as tiny calcifications, masses, or other changes that may not be felt during a clinical breast exam. The breast is compressed between two plates while an X-ray image is taken to detect abnormalities. It is recommended annually for women aged 40 or earlier for those with higher risk factors. As we know, cancer can evolve at earlier ages. This is why when starting puberty, it's important to do self-exams to know the normal look and feel of your breasts during your menstrual cycle and journal them. Mammograms can also detect cancerous changes at an early stage, often before they can be felt. Some breasts have discomfort from compression and the use of low-dose radiation.

Benefits of Breast Health

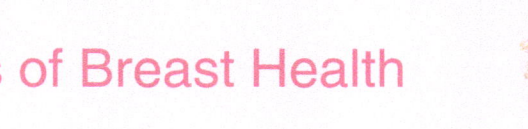

Thermography/Digital Imaging:

Thermography, or Digital Infrared Thermal Imaging (DITI), is a non-invasive, radiation-free screening method that measures the heat emitted from your body. It is beneficial for identifying abnormalities in breast health, as it can detect changes in blood flow and temperature patterns that may indicate the early stages of disease, including breast cancer.

These images reveal thermal patterns and hotspots that may indicate areas of concern. For breast health, thermography can detect changes in temperature and blood flow in the breast tissue. Increased heat can be an indicator of increased vascular activity, which could signal inflammation, hormonal imbalances, or, in some cases, the early stages of breast cancer.

While mammograms primarily detect structural changes (like lumps or tumors), thermography focuses on the physiological activity in breast tissue. This makes it ideal for identifying areas of inflammation or increased blood flow, which may occur before a tumor forms. It also helps assess breast health overall, detecting imbalances, infections, or hormonal fluctuations that can affect the breasts.

For women who prefer a more holistic approach to healthcare, thermography aligns with natural and preventative strategies.

While it should not replace mammograms, it can serve as a valuable complement, especially for younger women or those seeking a radiation-free option.

Benefits of Breast Health

Key Differences:

Self-breast exams, clinical exams, mammograms, and thermography each uniquely affect breast health. **Self-breast exams** involve regularly checking your own breasts for lumps or changes, promoting personal awareness but relying on touch alone. **Clinical breast exams**, performed by healthcare professionals, provide a more thorough hands-on examination for detecting abnormalities, though they may miss more minor changes not detectable by touch. **Mammograms** and breast X-ray imaging are the gold standard for early detection, identifying even tiny calcifications or tumors that cannot be felt. On the other hand, **Thermography** uses infrared imaging to detect heat patterns and blood flow changes that may indicate underlying issues.

While it is non-invasive and radiation-free, thermography should be used as a complementary tool rather than a replacement for mammograms, as it detects physiological rather than structural changes. Together, these methods offer a comprehensive approach to maintaining breast health.

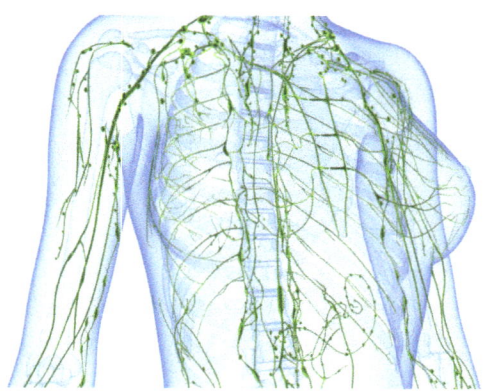

Benefits of Breast Health

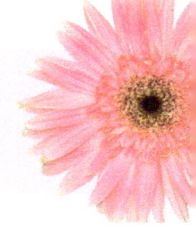

- **Prioritizing Breast Health:**

By prioritizing your breast health, you are taking a significant step toward your breast and your health. This includes scheduling regular check-ups with your healthcare provider, where they can perform clinical breast exams. During these visits, talking openly about your concerns and asking questions can help you understand what is happening with your body. Your doctor might also recommend mammograms or ultrasounds based on your age or family history, which are essential tools for early detection of potential issues

- **Healthy Habits:**

In addition to self-examinations and professional check-ups, adopting healthy habits can significantly benefit your breast health. A balanced diet of fruits, vegetables, and whole grains fuels your body with the necessary nutrients. Regular exercise is also vital, as it can help maintain a healthy weight and fatty tissue in the breast, which is essential for reducing the risk of breast conditions. Aim for at least 2.5 hours of moderate aerobic activity each week, such as brisk walking or cycling.

"Let's build wellness rather than treat disease."

Benefits of Breast Health

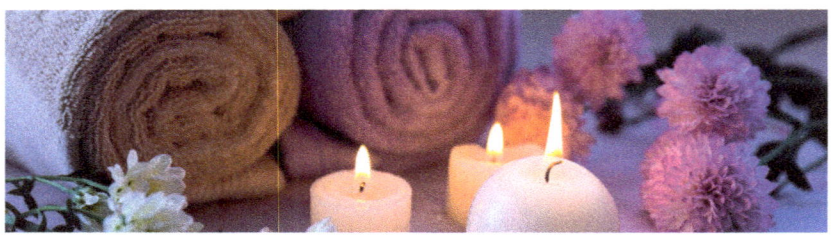

COMMON BREAST ISSUES

Several conditions can affect breast health, ranging from benign to malignant. Being aware of these conditions helps in recognizing symptoms and seeking timely medical attention.

Common Issues are:
- **Breast Cysts:** Fluid-filled sacs within the breast.
- **Breast Calcification:** are tiny deposits of calcium in the breast tissue.
- **Fibrocystic Changes:** Non-cancerous changes causing lumps or pain.
- **Mastitis:** Infection of the breast tissue, often during breastfeeding.
- **Post Surgical complication:** many may be benign and manageable, but some may require medical attention
- **Breast Cancer:** Malignant tumors that require prompt treatment.

Benefits of Breast Health

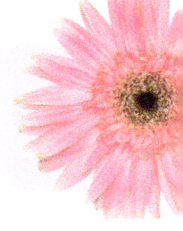

BREAST CYSTS

Breast cysts are fluid-filled structures within breast tissue that are usually benign, meaning they are not cancerous. These cysts are prevalent, particularly among women aged 35 to 50. Although they are mostly harmless, breast cysts can lead to physical discomfort and emotional anxiety. It is crucial to comprehend the characteristics of breast cysts, recognize their symptoms, and explore treatment options to ensure optimal breast health. These cysts can manifest as round or oval fluid-filled sacs, appearing in one or both breasts, and may range in size from microscopic, tiny formations to larger lumps when detected.

Types of Breast Cysts
- **Simple Cysts:**
    - These are thin, smooth-walled, fluid-filled sacs. They are usually benign and do not increase the risk of breast cancer.
- **Complex Cysts:**
    - These have both fluid and solid components. Although most complex cysts are benign, they may require further evaluation to rule out malignancy.

Benefits of Breast Health

BREAST CYSTS

Symptoms of Breast Cysts

- **Lump:** A smooth, easily movable lump in the breast that may feel tender or painful, especially before menstruation.
- **Breast Pain:** Pain or tenderness in the cyst area may fluctuate with the menstrual cycle.
- **Changes in Size:** The size and tenderness may also increase before the menstrual period and shrink afterward.
- **Nipple Discharge:** Rarely, cysts may cause clear or slightly cloudy nipple discharge.

Take note and journal these changes as they occur. Scheduling routine breast exams or imaging along with doing self-examination cysts can be discovered during these routine practices. The following diagnostic tools are commonly used:

- **Clinical Breast Exam:** A healthcare provider may feel a lump during a physical exam and recommend further testing.
- **Ultrasound:** ultrasounds can distinguish between solid masses and fluid-filled cysts.
- **Mammogram:** can help identify the size, the shape, and the location of cysts.

Benefits of Breast Health

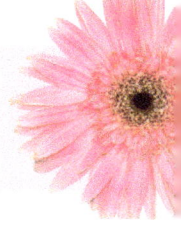

BREAST CYSTS

CAUSES OF BREAST CYST

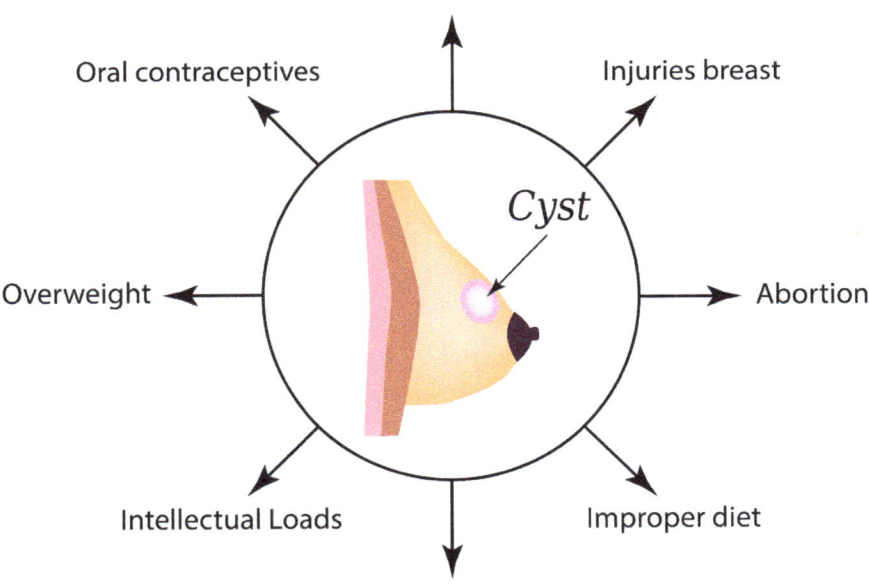

Benefits of Breast Health

BREAST CYSTS

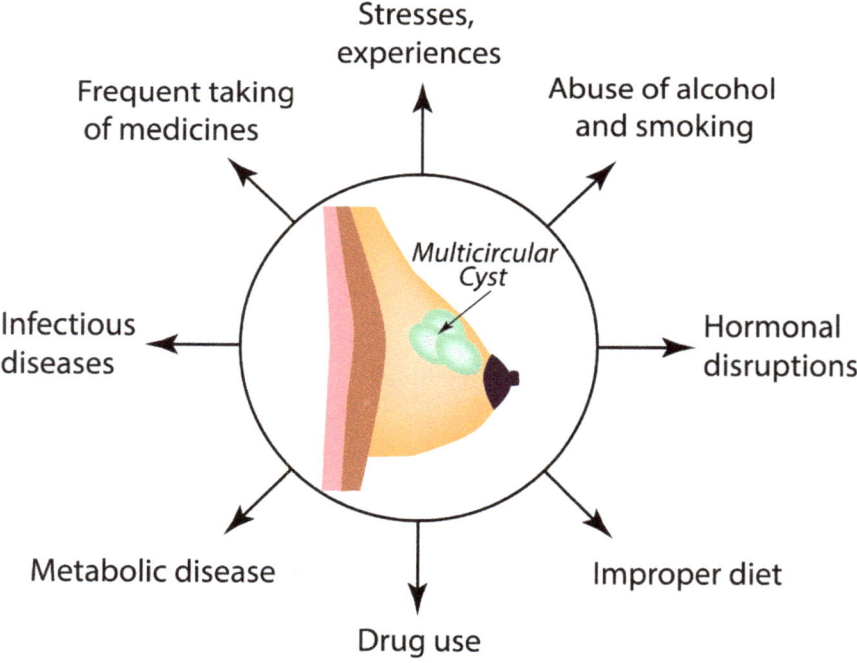

CAUSES OF MULTICIRCULAR CYST IN THE BREAST

- Stresses, experiences
- Abuse of alcohol and smoking
- Hormonal disruptions
- Improper diet
- Drug use
- Metabolic disease
- Infectious diseases
- Frequent taking of medicines

Multicircular Cyst

Benefits of Breast Health

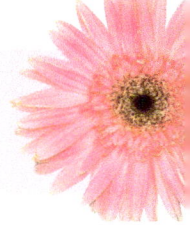

BREAST CYSTS

Simple Cysts that are not causing symptoms may be monitored with regular breast exams and imaging tests to ensure they do not change in size or character. If a cyst is painful or causing discomfort, a thin needle can drain the fluid. This procedure often provides immediate relief. It can help diagnose the cyst and relieve symptoms if the cyst is causing discomfort.

Cysts can be further evaluated or surgically removed if cysts become persistent, recurrent, or exhibit suspicious characteristics. Since most breast cysts are benign and do not require treatment, it is necessary to consult with your healthcare provider if you notice any new texture changes, such as alterations in breast size or shape, lumps, persistent tenderness or pain, skin changes like redness or dimpling, or nipple discharge—especially if blood is present without squeezing.

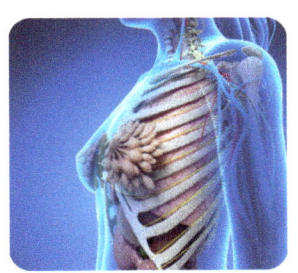

Benefits of Breast Health

FIBROCYSTIC TISSUE

When breast changes are prevalent due to texture and nodular appearance, this condition is called fibrocystic tissue. Although primarily benign, these changes impact many women, particularly those between the ages of 20 and 50. A thorough understanding of fibrocystic breast tissue can help alleviate worries and empower women to manage any symptoms they may encounter effectively.

Fibrocystic changes involve the development of fibrous tissue and cysts within the breast. This condition is often linked to hormonal shifts throughout the menstrual cycle, especially estrogen and progesterone. These hormonal variations can lead to lumpy, sensitive, and swollen breast tissue, particularly in the days leading up to menstruation.

It is crucial to notice and report any alterations in breast tissue to your healthcare provider promptly to exclude severe conditions. Diagnostic procedures are commonly followed to determine whether any growth is malignant or benign. These may include a mammogram or ultrasound, especially in younger individuals, as their breast tissue tends to be denser.

Due to this, an ultrasound is often preferred over a mammogram. Your healthcare provider will utilize these imaging techniques to assess the characteristics of the mass.

Benefits of Breast Health

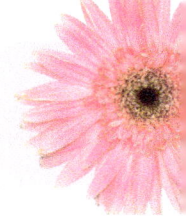

FIBROCYSTIC TISSUE

Characteristics

1. Lumps and Nodules:
- Cysts and fibrous tissue may cause the breast to feel lumpy or nodular. These lumps are usually movable and can vary in size.

2. Breast Pain and Tenderness:
- Women with fibrocystic changes often experience breast pain and tenderness, especially in the upper outer areas of the breast. The discomfort typically intensifies in the premenstrual phase.

3. Cysts:
- Cysts sacs that form in the breast tissue, can be small or large and may feel like round, movable lumps.

4. Fibrous Tissue:
- This refers to thickened, scar-like tissue within the breast, giving it a dense and firm texture.

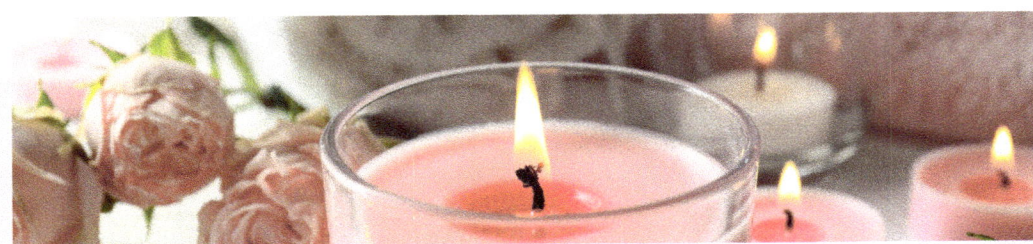

Benefits of Breast Health

FIBROCYSTIC TISSUE

Fibrocystic Care

1. Self-Care:
- Wearing a supportive bra reduces breast movement and discomfort of the fibrocystic tissue.
- Using Castor Oil packs can increase blood flow and decrease inflammation in fibrocystic breasts.
- Applying warm or cold compresses to alleviate pain and swelling.
- Over-the-counter pain relievers can help manage pain.

2. Lifestyle Modifications:
- Reducing caffeine intake, as some women have stated that caffeine has worsened their symptoms.
- Eating a balanced diet rich in fruits, vegetables, and whole grains can be supportive.
- Maintaining a healthy weight and exercising regularly to promote hormonal balance.

3. Medical Treatments:
- In severe cases, hormonal therapies or prescription medications may be recommended by a healthcare provider.
- Aspiration, a fluid drainage procedure from large, painful cysts, can provide relief.

Benefits of Breast Health

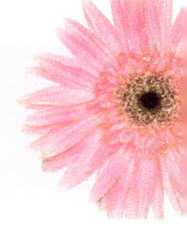

FIBROCYSTIC TISSUE

WHEN TO SEEK ATTENTION

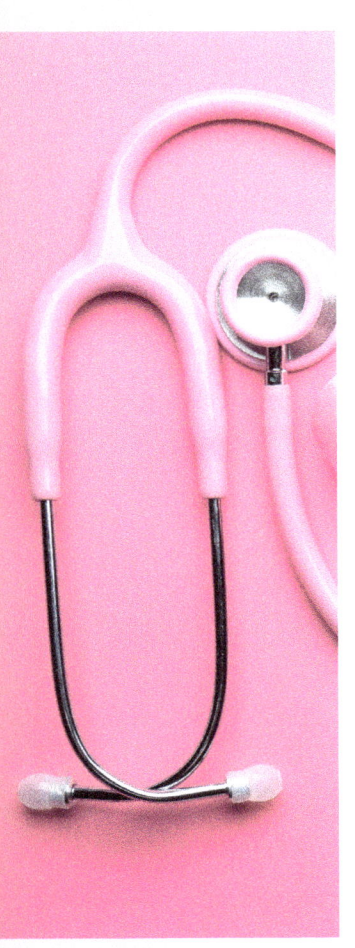

While fibrocystic changes are generally benign, it is essential to monitor any changes in your breasts and consult a healthcare provider if you notice:

- New or unusual lumps that persist after your menstrual cycle.

- Changes in the size, shape, or appearance of your breasts.

- Nipple discharge, particularly bloody. Persistent or severe pain that does not improve with self-care measures.

Benefits of Breast Health

BREAST CALCIFICATION

Breast calcifications are tiny deposits of calcium that appear within the breast tissue. These calcifications are usually detected on a mammogram as small white spots or flecks and are common in women, especially after menopause.

While they are generally benign (non-cancerous), specific patterns may indicate the presence of breast cancer or other medical issues, warranting further examination.

How Do Breast Calcifications Happen?
Breast calcifications occur when calcium builds up in the breast tissue. The exact cause of this buildup is not always clear, but several factors can contribute to the development of calcifications:

1. Aging: Calcifications are more common in older women, particularly after menopause.

2. Previous Injuries or Infections: Trauma or inflammation in the breast tissue, such as surgery, injury, or radiation therapy, can lead to calcification.

Benefits of Breast Health

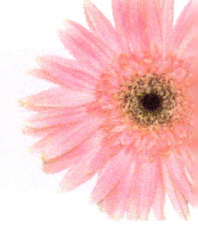

BREAST CALCIFICATION

3. Benign Breast Conditions: Conditions like fibrocystic changes, fibroadenomas, or benign cysts can sometimes lead to calcifications.

4. Calcium Deposits in Blood Vessels: Sometimes, calcium deposits can occur in the blood vessels of the breast, which is generally unrelated to breast cancer.

5. Ductal Changes: Calcifications can form in the milk ducts due to secretions, dead cells, or ductal hyperplasia (an overgrowth of cells within the ducts).

CALCIFICATIONS IN THE BREAST

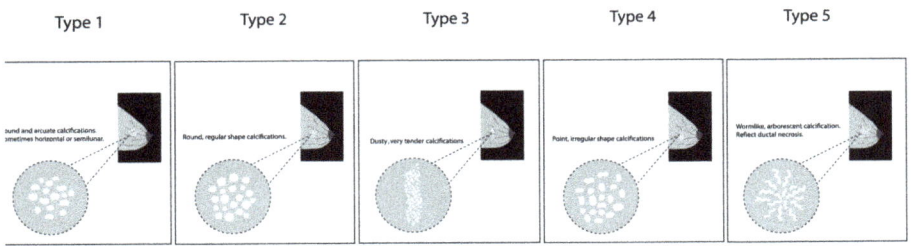

Benefits of Breast Health

BREAST CALCIFICATION

There are two types of Breast Calcifications.

Breast calcifications are generally categorized into two types:

1. Macrocalcifications: These are larger, coarse calcium deposits usually associated with benign conditions. They are common, especially in women over 50, and are not usually linked to cancer.

2. Microcalcifications: These are tiny calcium deposits that can appear in clusters. While they are often benign, specific patterns of microcalcifications can indicate early breast cancer or precancerous changes, such as ductal carcinoma in situ (DCIS).

When calcifications are detected on a mammogram, their appearance is carefully analyzed by a radiologist. If the calcifications are deemed suspicious, additional imaging, such as magnification views, may be performed to get a closer look. If further evaluation is needed, a biopsy might be recommended to determine if the calcifications are associated with cancer.

Benefits of Breast Health

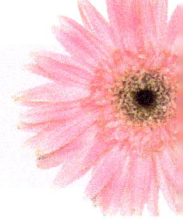

BREAST CALCIFICATION

The treatment approach depends on the nature of the calcifications and the underlying cause:

1. Benign Calcifications:
- Observation: If the calcifications are benign, no treatment is needed. Routine mammograms may be recommended to monitor any changes over time.

2. Suspicious or Malignant Calcifications:
- Biopsy: If the calcifications are suspicious, a biopsy is performed to determine whether cancer is present. This may be done using a needle (core needle biopsy) or through surgical excision.

- Surgery: If cancer or precancerous cells are found, surgery might be necessary to remove the affected tissue. This could involve a lumpectomy (removal of the tumor and some surrounding tissue) or a mastectomy (removal of the entire breast), depending on the extent of the disease.

- Radiation Therapy: If the calcifications are associated with early-stage breast cancer, radiation therapy may be recommended after surgery to reduce the risk of recurrence.

- Hormonal Therapy: Hormonal therapy might be used to block the effects of estrogen on breast cancer cells.

Benefits of Breast Health

BREAST CALCIFICATION

3. **Management of Underlying Conditions:**
   - Treatment of Infections or Injuries: If calcifications are related to previous infections or injuries, treatment may focus on managing these underlying conditions.

Follow-Up and Prevention

Regular mammograms and follow-up imaging are crucial for women with a history of breast calcifications, particularly if they have been associated with suspicious or malignant findings. Preventive measures for breast health include maintaining a healthy lifestyle, regular self-exams, and routine screenings as recommended by healthcare providers.

Breast calcifications are generally not a cause for alarm, but understanding their nature and the importance of monitoring
them is key to maintaining breast health. If further evaluation is needed, a biopsy might be recommended to determine if the calcifications are associated with cancer.

Benefits of Breast Health

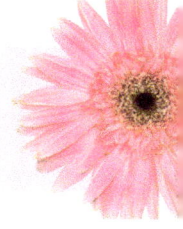

BREAST CALCIFICATION

Understanding Breast Calcifications and Lymphatic Drainage reveals that breast tissue does not directly interact with lymphatic fluid flow. The primary objective of lymphatic drainage is to facilitate the movement of lymph fluid, alleviate swelling, and promote detoxification; however, lymph flow does not impact the formation of calcium deposits within the breast tissue.

The occurrence of calcifications is predominantly influenced by variables such as aging, previous injuries, infections, or benign breast conditions rather than any complications related to lymphatic fluid movement.

Providing Lymphatic Drainage massage can simply impact the surrounding tissue, while modalities such as myofascial and breast massage can keep non-calcified tissue in a healthier state.

Benefits of Breast Health

BREAST MASTITIS

Mastitis is inflammation of the breast tissue that can result in warmth, redness, swelling, and pain. It is most commonly associated with breastfeeding but can also occur in women who are not breastfeeding and, in rare cases, in men. Understanding mastitis, its causes, symptoms, and treatment options is essential for maintaining breast health and preventing complications.

Mastitis is often caused by a bacterial infection that enters the breast tissue through a cracked or sore nipple. It typically affects breastfeeding women, especially within the first few weeks after childbirth. The condition can lead to the development of a swollen and painful area in the breast and, if left untreated, may sometimes result in an abscess.

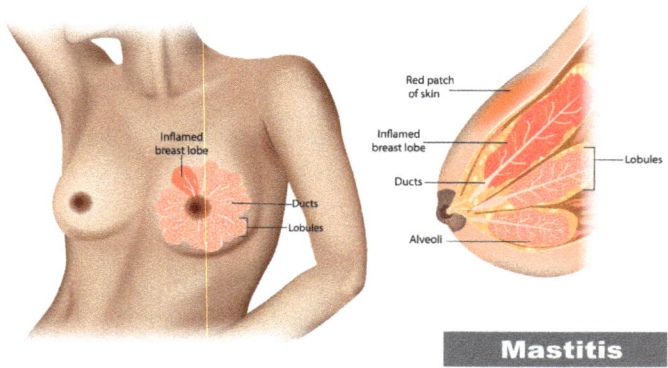

Benefits of Breast Health

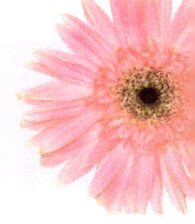

BREAST MASTITIS

1. **Bacterial Infection:**
   - The most common cause of mastitis is a bacterial infection. Bacteria from the skin's surface or the baby's mouth can enter the breast tissue through cracks in the nipple.

2. **Blocked Milk Ducts:**
   - When a milk duct becomes blocked, milk can back up and lead to infection. This can occur if a baby is not correctly latching onto the breast or breastfeeding sessions are infrequent.

3. **Weakened Immune System:**
   - Due to stress, fatigue, or illness, a weakened immune system can make a woman more susceptible to infections, including mastitis.

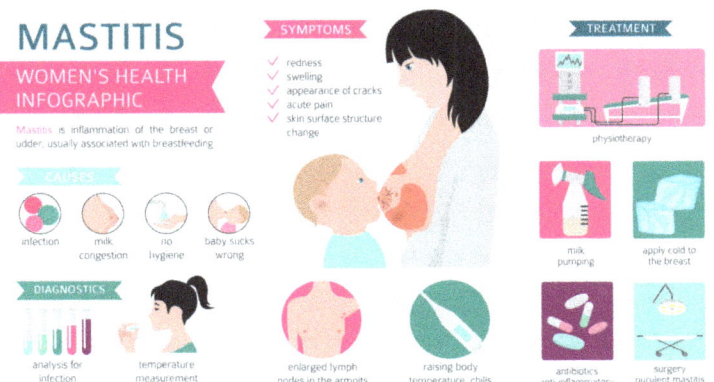

Benefits of Breast Health

BREAST MASTITIS

Symptoms of Mastitis

- **Breast Pain:** Sharp or shooting pain in one or both breasts.

- **Swelling:** Noticeable swelling in the affected breast.

- **Redness and Warmth**: The breast may appear red and feel warm.

- **Fever and Chills:** Mastitis often causes flu-like symptoms, including fever and chills.
- **Fatigue:** A general feeling of tiredness and malaise.

- **Nipple Discharge:** Pus or other discharge from the nipple.

A healthcare provider can diagnose mastitis based on a physical examination and the patient's symptoms. Sometimes, a breast milk sample may be tested to identify the type of bacteria causing the infection.

Benefits of Breast Health

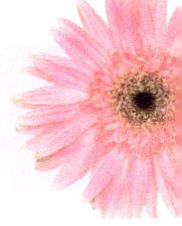

BREAST MASTITIS

Bacterial Mastitis is primarily treated with antibiotics. Completing your prescribed course of antibiotics is essential to eradicate the infection. Over-the-counter pain relievers, such as ibuprofen, can also effectively alleviate pain and minimize inflammation.

Continuing to breastfeed or express milk remains vital, even in the face of discomfort. This encourages milk flow and helps prevent additional blockages. Implementing proper latch techniques and feeding frequently can speed up recovery. The use of warm compresses on the affected breast can also ease pain and enhance milk flow; a warm, damp washcloth or a heating pad can serve this purpose well.

Rest and adequate hydration are crucial for healing. Prioritizing rest and fluid intake strengthens the body's ability to combat the infection more efficiently.

TREATMENT

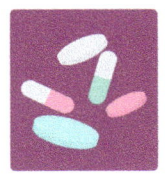
antibiotics
anti-inflammatory

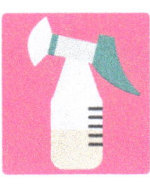
milk
pumping

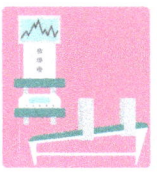
physiotherapy

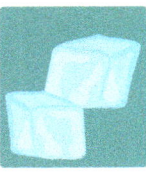
apply cold to
the breast

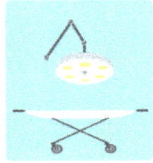
surgery
purulent mastitis

Benefits of Breast Health

BREAST MASTITIS

Preventing Mastitis

- Proper Breastfeeding Techniques: Ensure the baby is latching correctly and feeding frequently to prevent milk stasis.

- Nipple Care: Keep the nipples clean and dry, and use nipple creams if needed to prevent cracking.

- Avoid Tight Bras: Wear comfortable, well-fitting bras that do not constrict the breasts during breastfeeding.

- Hand Hygiene: Wash hands regularly, especially before breastfeeding, to reduce the risk of infection.

Seek Medical Attention: if you experience symptoms of mastitis, it is essential to seek medical attention as soon as possible. Early treatment can prevent complications such as abscess formation. Contact a healthcare provider if you notice severe breast pain or swelling, persistent fever or flu-like symptoms, pus or unusual discharge from the nipple, and symptoms that do not improve within 24-48 hours of home treatment.

Benefits of Breast Health

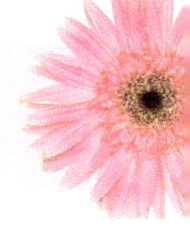

POST SURGICAL CONDITIONS

Plastic breast surgeries, such as augmentation, reduction, or reconstruction, are standard procedures that can lead to various postoperative conditions. While many of these conditions are benign and manageable, some may require medical attention. Here are some common breast conditions that may arise after breast surgical procedures:

1.   **Capsular Contracture:** Contracture occurs when scar tissue (a capsule) that naturally forms around a breast implant squeezes, tightens, and compresses the implant. This type of compression can cause the breast to feel firm and uncomfortable, develop hardness, and distort the shape of the breast, causing much pain. Some treatment options may include breast massages to help loosen tightness around the implant and soften the tissue, medication, or surgery to remove or replace the implant and scar tissue.

2.   **Hematoma:** A hematoma is a collection of blood outside blood vessels that can occur after surgery due to bleeding. Symptoms often include swelling, bruising, pain, and a feeling of fullness in the breast. Small hematomas may resolve independently, but larger ones might require drainage or surgical intervention.

Benefits of Breast Health

POST SURGICAL CONDITIONS

3. Seroma: A seroma is a fluid buildup in the tissue surrounding the surgical site. This is more common after extensive procedures like breast reconstruction. Symptoms of seromas include swelling, fluid-filled pockets under the skin, discomfort, and a feeling of fullness. Depending on the size and symptoms, seromas may be drained with a needle or left to absorb naturally. Massage should be minimal in that area until draining with a needle is no longer needed. Massaging when draining is required can lead to more oversized pockets or develop more than one seroma.

4. Infections: can occur at the surgical site, around the implants, or in the breast tissue after surgery. Check for redness, warmth, swelling, pain, fever, and drainage from the incision site. Typically, you may require antibiotics, and in some cases, you may have additional surgery.

5. Changes in Sensation: Numbness, hypersensitivity, or loss of sensation in the breast or nipple area can occur and be expected after surgery due to nerve damage. Symptoms include numbness, tingling, increased sensitivity, or a complete loss of feeling in the breast or nipple. These sensation changes often improve over time as nerves heal, but some changes may be permanent.

Benefits of Breast Health

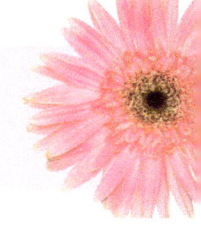

POST SURGICAL CONDITIONS

6. Asymmetry refers to visible unevenness between the two breasts in size, shape, or position, which can occur after surgery. It's important to wait until swelling and inflammation have decreased to see true asymmetry, at which point revision surgery may be required to correct significant asymmetry.

7. Breast Implant Rupture: Breast implants can rupture or leak, particularly in older implants or those that have undergone trauma. You could experience a sudden change in breast shape or size, lumps, pain, or asymmetry. The rupture might be "faint" and not immediately noticeable in silicone implants. It may be necessary for the removal or replacement of the implant.

8. Breast Ptosis (Sagging): Breast sagging can occur over time, especially after augmentation or reduction surgery, due to aging, gravity, and changes in weight. You may consider a breast lift (mastopexy) later to correct this significant sagging.

Benefits of Breast Health

POST SURGICAL CONDITIONS

9. Fat Necrosis: occurs when fat tissue in the breast becomes damaged and forms firm lumps. This can happen after breast reconstruction, reduction, or augmentation, especially in cases where fat transfer and fat grafting are involved. Fat necrosis can lead to firm lumps, pain, or changes in breast shape. They are usually benign and may resolve on their own, but in some cases, these lumps may need to be removed surgically because of discomfort or are mistaken for cancer.

10. Scarring: All surgeries result in some scarring, but the extent can vary. Some individuals may develop hypertrophic scars or keloids, which are raised, thickened scars. Scar massage treatments, steroid injections, laser therapy, or revision surgery can minimize scar tissue.

11. Breast Pain (Mastalgia): Pain is also widespread after any surgical procedure, including breast surgery, due to healing, swelling, or nerve irritation. Pain may include Tenderness, sharp pain, or a dull ache in the breast. Applying cold compresses, comfortable bras, pain relievers, and light breast massages can alleviate some discomfort.

Benefits of Breast Health

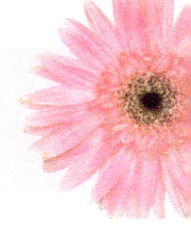

POST SURGICAL CONDITIONS

12. Lymphedema: Lymphedema is swelling caused by lymphatic fluid buildup, which can occur in the arm or breast after removing lymph node(s), radiation therapy during breast reconstruction, or other breast surgeries. Lymphodema is swelling of fluid, heaviness, or tightness in the affected area. Lymphedema management includes a combination of compression garments, physical therapy, and manual lymphatic drainage massages.

13. Rippling: Breast rippling refers to the visible or palpable folds or wrinkles in the breast implant, often felt under the skin, especially in women with thin breast tissue. This can be treated with adjustments such as adding more tissue coverage or replacing the implant may be considered.

Many of these conditions are manageable, and the likelihood of serious complications can be minimized with surgeons with good surgical techniques and knowledgeable postoperative care. It's essential to follow your surgeon's advice, attend all follow-up appointments, and promptly report any unusual changes or symptoms to your healthcare provider. Monitoring your healing and a healthy lifestyle can help ensure the best outcomes after breast surgery.

Benefits of Breast Health

BREAST CANCER IDENTIFIERS

Recognizing the symptoms of breast cancer early is crucial for breast health, effective treatments, and better outcomes. While some people may not experience any symptoms in the early stages, several signs and symptoms could indicate the presence of breast cancer.

A new lump or mass in the breast is one of the most common symptoms of breast cancer. It can feel like a hard, painless lump with irregular edges, but breast cancer lumps can also be soft, rounded, and tender. Any new lump or mass should be evaluated by a healthcare provider, even if it is painless.

Any unexplained change in the breast's size, shape, or contour could be a warning sign; this includes swelling of all or part of the breast (even if no distinct lump is felt). Breast cancer can cause changes in the appearance of the nipples, including a newly inverted (pulled in) nipple and unusual nipple discharge, mainly if it is clear, bloody, or occurs without squeezing, redness, scaling, or thickening of the nipple or areola (the dark area surrounding the nipple). Take action if you notice any nipple changes, mainly if they are new or unusual, and consult a healthcare provider.

Benefits of Breast Health

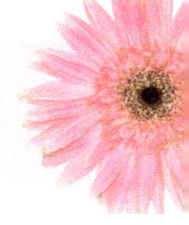

BREAST CANCER IDENTIFIERS

Breast cancer can also cause changes in the skin over the breast, such as dimpling or puckering, which may resemble the surface of an orange peel or show different textures compared to the normal appearance and feel of the breast. Additionally, if you notice any surrounding tissue that feels unusually warm to the touch, touch and feel your breast to see if the skin has become thickened or feels differently to the touch. Persistent or unusual pain should not be ignored. Persistent redness or a rash on the breast can be a sign of inflammatory breast cancer, a rare but aggressive form of the disease.

Swelling or lumps in the armpit can indicate that cancer has spread to the lymph nodes in the area, causing these symptoms. Such lumps may be felt even before a tumor is detected in the breast. Additionally, breast pain after menopause is less common; thus, new pain in one or both breasts could be a sign of a problem.

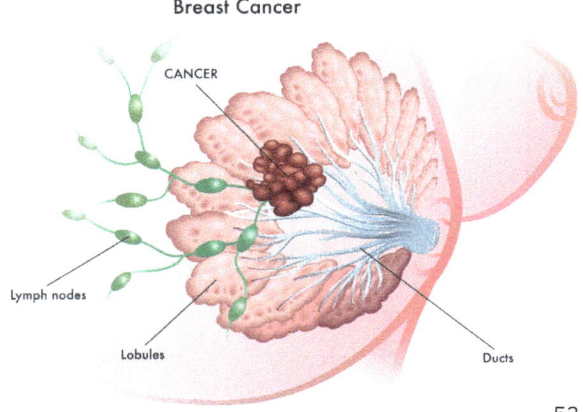

Benefits of Breast Health

BREAST CANCER IDENTIFIERS

Even though these are more general symptoms, unexplained weight loss or persistent fatigue can sometimes be associated with advanced breast cancer. If you experience significant weight loss or fatigue without a clear cause, please make sure you make an appointment to discuss these symptoms with your healthcare provider.

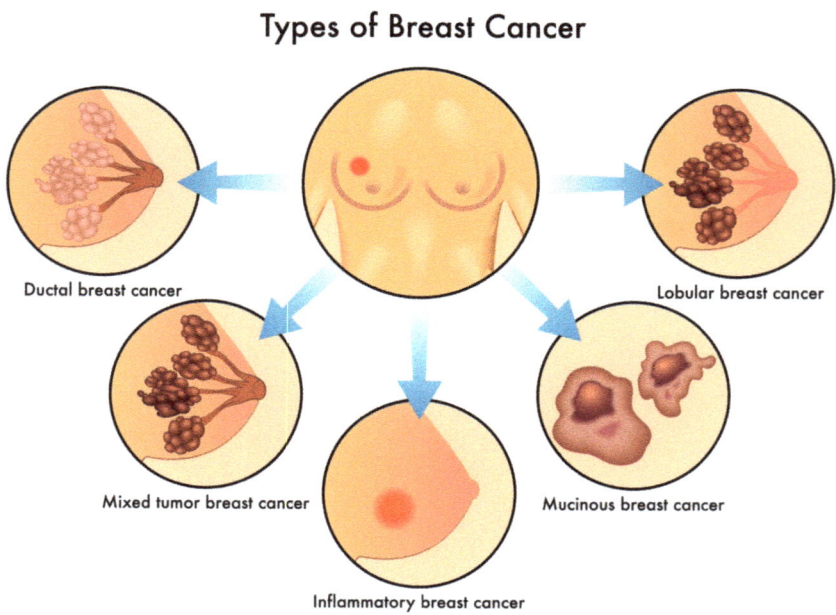

Chapter 3
The Role of Lymphatic Breast Health

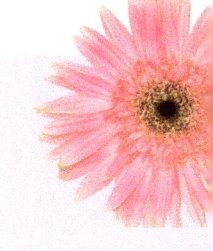

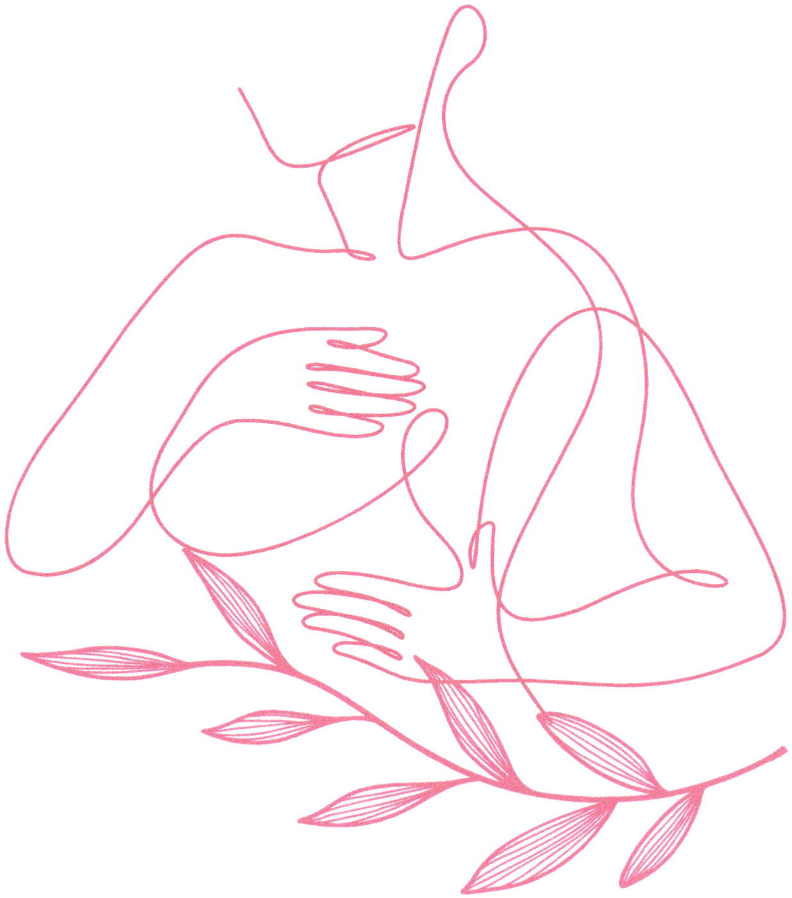

Role of Lymphatic Breast Health

LYMPHATIC BREAST HEALTH

Understanding the physiology of the lymphatic system in the breast is essential for appreciating how it contributes to breast health. The lymphatic system plays a crucial role in maintaining fluid balance, filtering out harmful substances, and supporting immune function. This chapter explores the structure and function of the lymphatic system within the breast, highlighting its importance and physiological processes.

The lymphatic system in the breast consists of lymphatic vessels, lymph nodes, and lymph fluid. These components work together to transport and filter lymph, a clear fluid that contains white blood cells, proteins, and waste products.

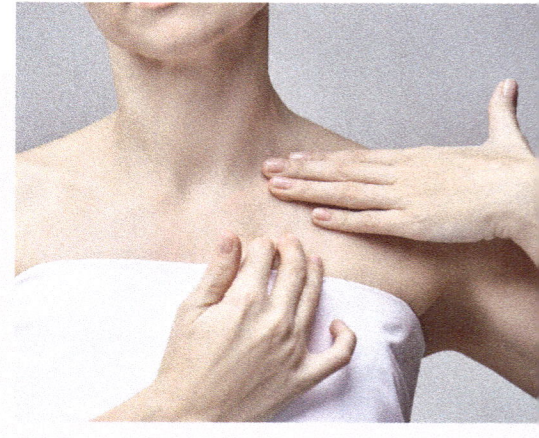

"Massage is a therapy that speaks the language of the body."

Role of Lymphatic Breast Health

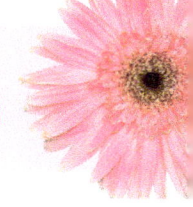

LYMPHATIC BREAST HEALTH

Lymphatic Components:

1. **Lymphatic Vessels:**
   - These are thin, walled tubes that collect and transport lymph fluid. They begin as small capillaries that converge into larger vessels, eventually draining into lymph nodes.
2. **Lymph Nodes:**
   - Small, bean-shaped structures that filter lymph fluid, removing bacteria, viruses, and other harmful substances. The breast contains several lymph nodes, primarily located in the axillary (armpit) region, as well as the internal mammary (breast) and supraclavicular (collarbone) regions.
3. **Lymph Fluid:**
   - A clear, colorless fluid that circulates through the lymphatic vessels. It contains lymphocytes (white blood cells), proteins, and waste products from cellular processes.

Role of Lymphatic Breast Health

LYMPHATIC BREAST HEALTH

This system is crucial for our immunity because it transports lymph fluid, which contains white blood cells that help fight infection and other substances that need to be filtered and removed from the body. In the breasts, the lymphatic system helps maintain tissue health and prevent congestion.

The following functions show the physiology of the lymphatic system:

Fluid Balance:
The lymphatic system helps maintain fluid balance by collecting excess interstitial fluid (the fluid surrounding cells) and returning it to the bloodstream. This process prevents the buildup of excess fluid, which can lead to swelling and edema, making the breast feel fuller and heavier than usual.

Immune Response:
Lymph nodes act as filtering stations that trap and destroy pathogens such as bacteria, viruses, and abnormal cells. Lymphocytes within the nodes identify and attack these foreign invaders, which is crucial to the body's immune defense.

Role of Lymphatic Breast Health

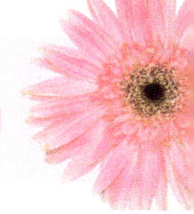

LYMPHATIC BREAST HEALTH

Waste Removal:

The lymphatic system transports waste products, cellular debris, and toxins away from the tissues and toward the lymph nodes for filtration. This process aids in detoxification and helps maintain healthy breast tissue.

Lymphatic drainage in the breast primarily occurs through three main pathways:

1. **Axillary (armpit) Pathway:**
   - Most breast lymph fluid drains towards the axillary lymph nodes in the armpits. This primary drainage route is crucial for filtering lymph from the outer and central parts of the breast.
   -

2. **Internal Mammary (breast) Pathway:**
   - Some lymph fluid drains towards the internal mammary lymph nodes located along the sternum (breastbone). This pathway is important for draining lymph from the inner parts of the breast.

Role of Lymphatic Breast Health

LYMPHATIC BREAST HEALTH

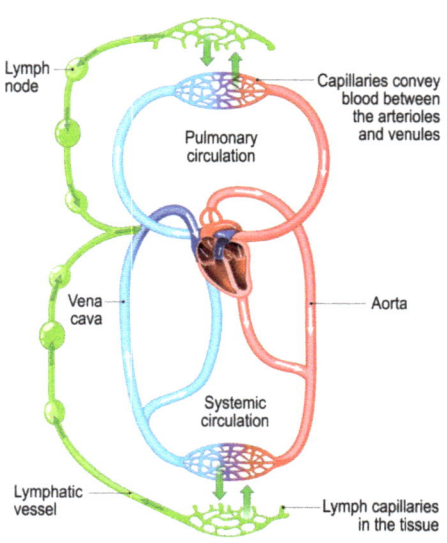

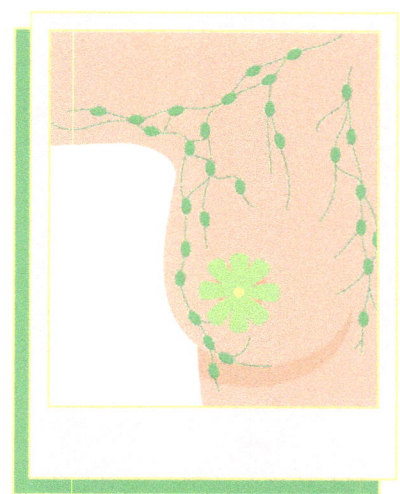

Role of Lymphatic Breast Health

LYMPHATIC BREAST HEALTH

3. **Supraclavicular Pathway:**
   - A smaller amount of lymph fluid drains towards the supraclavicular (above collarbone) lymph nodes, which are located above the collarbone. This pathway assists in draining lymph from the upper parts of the breast.

Physiological Processes in Lymphatic Drainage

Lymph Formation:

- Lymph fluid is formed when interstitial fluid (fluid in vessels), which surrounds the cells in the breast tissue, enters the lymphatic capillaries. This fluid contains nutrients, oxygen, and waste products from cellular metabolism.

Lymph Transport:

- Lymph fluid is transported through the lymphatic vessels by a combination of smooth muscle contractions, the contraction of surrounding skeletal muscles, and one-way valves that prevent backflow. This process ensures the continuous movement of lymph towards the lymph nodes.

Role of Lymphatic Breast Health

LYMPHATIC BREAST HEALTH

Lymph Filtration:
- As lymph fluid passes through the lymph nodes, it is filtered to remove pathogens, debris, and abnormal cells. Lymphocytes within the nodes identify and attack these foreign substances, preventing them from entering the bloodstream.

Lymphatic Return:
- Filtered lymph fluid is eventually returned to the bloodstream through the thoracic duct or the right lymphatic duct, which empties into the subclavian veins. This process maintains fluid balance and ensures the proper circulation of immune cells and nutrients.

It is important to understand how a healthy lymphatic system is vital for maintaining breast health and preventing various conditions. Providing self-care massages and seeking professional routine lymphatic drainage massages can significantly aid in your ongoing breast care. Efficient lymphatic drainage helps reduce the risk of infections, lymphedema (swelling due to lymph fluid buildup), and the accumulation of toxins that can damage breast tissue.

Chapter 4
Holistic Approach to Breast Health

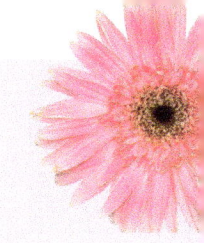

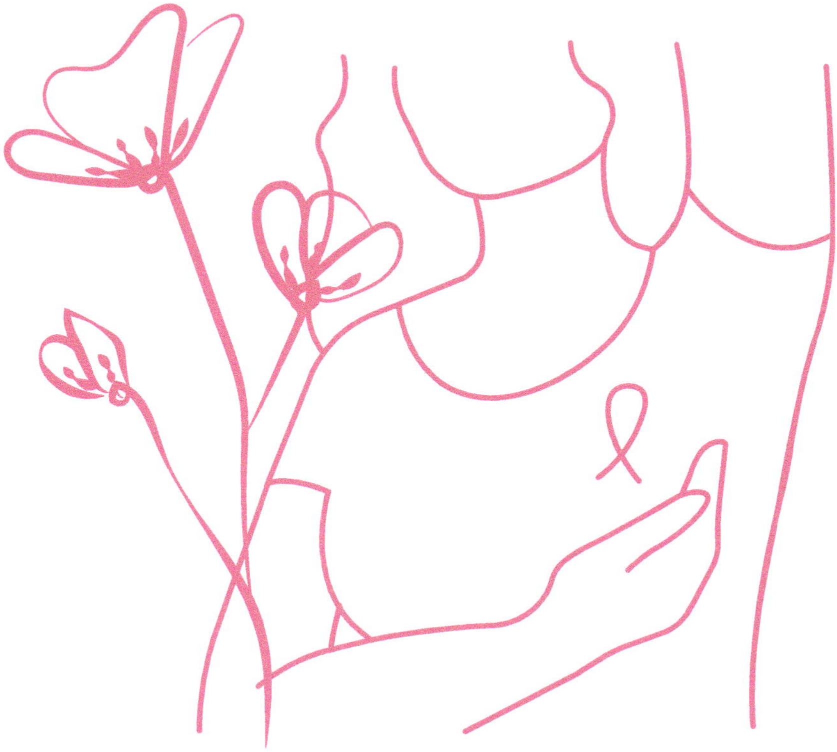

Holistic Approach to Breast Health

HOLISTIC APPROACHES

Maintaining Breast Health is a multifaceted endeavor that significantly benefits from combining traditional medical practices and holistic approaches. Lymphatic drainage massage, in particular, is a powerful tool for promoting breast health, complemented by various holistic strategies that support breast wellness.

Lymphatic Drainage Massage is a therapeutic technique designed to enhance the flow of lymph fluid. Understanding how lymphatic drainage massage works and its specific benefits can empower women to incorporate this practice into their regular self-care.

Breast lymphatic drainage massage is benefited by:

- Reduces swelling and fluid retention.
- Enhances immunity.
- Detoxification.
- Improve circulation.
- Pain and discomfort.

Holistic Approach to Breast Health

HOLISTIC APPROACHES

Massage Therapy is essential for breast health, whether it's done by a therapist or through self-care. Both methods contribute uniquely to better lymphatic flow.

1. **Reduces Swelling and Fluid Retention**

Lymphatic drainage massage can help reduce swelling and fluid retention in the breasts, which are often caused by hormonal changes, injury, or surgery. By promoting the flow of lymphatic fluid, this massage technique helps drain excess fluid from the breast tissue, reducing discomfort and swelling.

2. **Enhances Immune Function**

Lymphatic drainage massage stimulates the lymphatic system on a greater level when manually stimulated and supports the body's immune function. Improved lymphatic circulation enhances the removal of toxins and waste products, which can help prevent infections and support overall breast health. Maintaining immune health is crucial; if breast cancer occurs, a robust immune system can help fight off infections, supported by healthy liver function.

Holistic Approach to Breast Health

HOLISTIC APPROACHES

3. Promotes Detoxification

The detoxification process facilitates the removal of metabolic waste and toxins from the breast tissue. This can help maintain healthy breast tissue and prevent the buildup of potentially harmful substances. Overall, the shape of the breast can be more fluid, balanced, and visually symmetric.

4. Improves Circulation

Enhancing circulation can support tissue repair and regeneration, promoting breast health. Massaging the breast improves blood and lymph circulation, ensuring nutrients and oxygen are efficiently delivered to the breast tissue.

5. Relieves Pain and Discomfort

Lymphatic drainage massage alleviates pain and discomfort associated with fibrocystic breast changes, lymphedema, and post-surgical recovery. The gentle, rhythmic movements help reduce pressure and tenderness in the breast tissue. Some clients have restricted arm movements, and pain-providing fascia release can greatly improve arm and shoulder rotation.

Holistic Approach to Breast Health

HOLISTIC APPROACHES

Acupuncture

Acupuncture is a traditional Chinese medicine practice that can help balance hormones, reduce inflammation, and improve lymphatic circulation. It is often used to address issues like hormonal imbalances, pain, and swelling.

- How It Works: Acupuncture involves the insertion of fine needles into specific points on the body to stimulate energy flow (qi) and support overall health.

Castor Oil Packs

Castor oil packs are an ancient remedy for reducing inflammation and promoting lymphatic flow. Castor oil contains ricinoleic acid, which has anti-inflammatory and detoxifying properties.

How to Use: Soak a cotton cloth in castor oil, place it over the breast area, and cover it with plastic wrap or light cloth as a barrier. Apply a moist heating pad (moist heat is better than dry) or hot water bottle on top for 20-30 minutes. This helps promote circulation and lymphatic drainage in the breast tissue.

Holistic Approach to Breast Health

HOLISTIC APPROACHES

Thermal Therapy (Far Infrared Saunas)

Far infrared saunas use gentle heat to promote detoxification, improve circulation, and support the lymphatic system. The increased sweating helps the body eliminate toxins, while the heat boosts circulation, which can benefit breast tissue and overall health.

Hydrotherapy:

Hydrotherapy, or alternating hot and cold water, can stimulate circulation and lymphatic movement.

- Contrast Showers: Alternating between hot and cold water in the shower can improve circulation and stimulate the lymphatic system. This helps flush toxins and reduce swelling in the breast tissue.
- Warm Baths with Epsom Salt: Epsom salts contain magnesium, which can help reduce inflammation and promote detoxification.

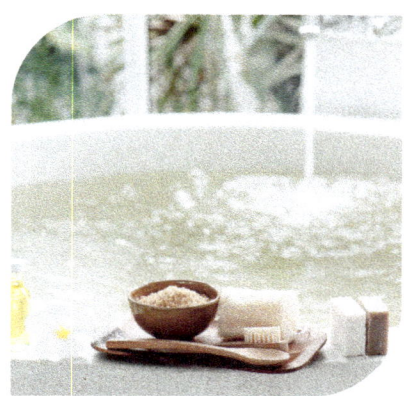

Holistic Approach to Breast Health

HOLISTIC APPROACHES

Herbal Remedies

Certain herbs have properties that support hormonal balance, reduce inflammation, and promote breast health.

Turmeric: This powerful anti-inflammatory herb may help prevent the growth of abnormal cells and reduce inflammation in breast tissue.

Milk Thistle: Known for supporting liver detoxification, milk thistle helps remove toxins from the body that could affect breast health.

Red Clover: Contains phytoestrogens, which may help balance hormone levels and support healthy breast tissue.

Dandelion Root: Acts as a detoxifying agent, promoting healthy liver function and lymphatic drainage.

Green Tea: Rich in antioxidants, particularly catechins, green tea has been linked to a reduced risk of breast cancer.

Essential Oils and Aromatherapy

- Essential oils like lavender, frankincense, and rose have anti-inflammatory and relaxing properties that may support breast health. These oils can be applied topically (when diluted with a carrier oil) or used in aromatherapy to help relieve stress and promote relaxation, which is beneficial for overall health and hormonal balance.
- Clary sage and geranium oils can help regulate hormone levels, particularly estrogen, which can impact breast health and PMS symptoms.

Holistic Approach to Breast Health

HOLISTIC APPROACHES

Mind-Body Practices:

Mind-body practices can reduce stress and enhance emotional well-being, benefiting overall breast health. Journaling and writing down thoughts and feelings can help reduce stress and improve mental health. A tapping technique known as emotional freedom therapy can help reduce emotional stress, which may impact stress reduction and nerve stimulation, as well as breast health.

Holistic therapies for breast health focus on nurturing the body's natural healing abilities and maintaining balance. By integrating these practices into your lifestyle, you can support your breast and lymphatic health, enhance detoxification, and promote overall wellness. Always consult with a healthcare provider to ensure these therapies are safe and appropriate for your individual needs.

Chapter 5
Lymphatic Massage Techniques

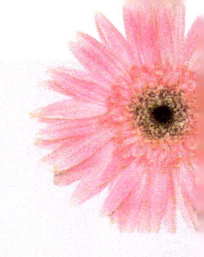

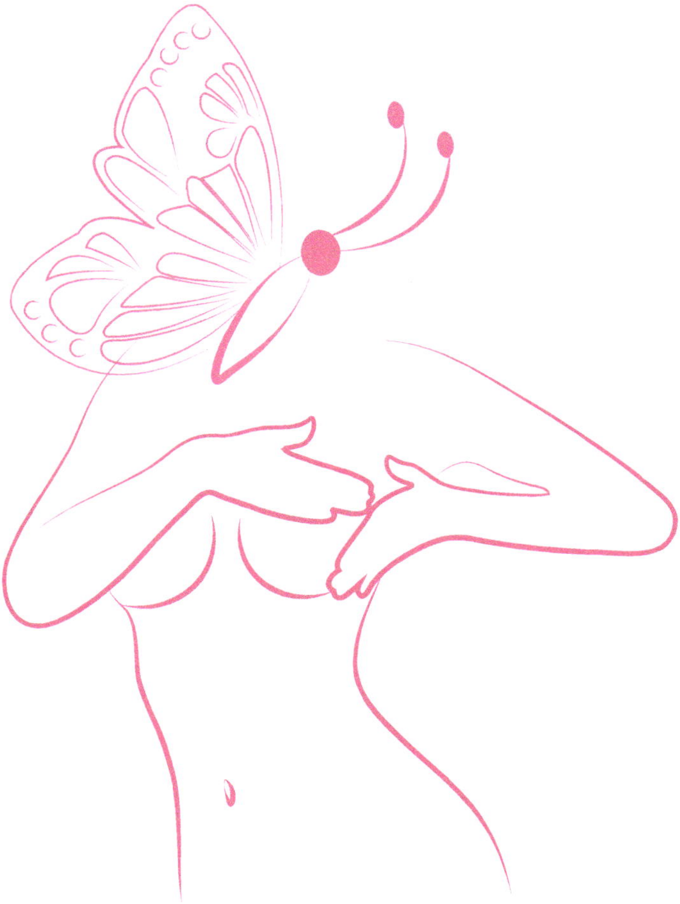

Lymphatic Massage Techniques

LYMPHATIC MASSAGES

Several techniques can be used to promote lymphatic drainage, including Manual Lymphatic Drainage (MLD), Myofascial Release, Gentle Breast Massages, Exercise, and Proper Hydration.

These techniques help keep the breast soft and supple and maintain natural lymphatic flow, which can sometimes be disrupted by the prolonged use of restrictive bras that encase the breast and inhibit natural flow. Breasts should be allowed to 'breathe' periodically to promote healthy circulation.

Drink plenty of water, not just for your breasts but to keep the body hydrated regularly for full-body lymphatic flow.

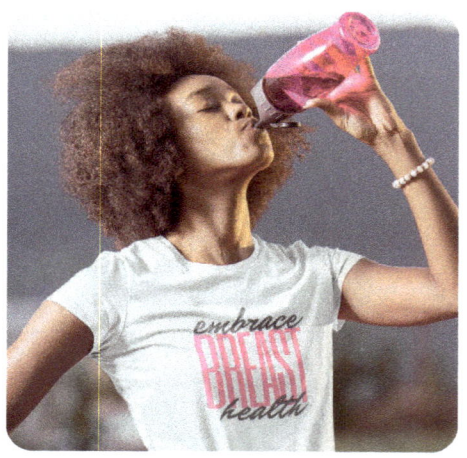

Lymphatic Massage Techniques

LYMPHATIC MASSAGES

Manual Lymphatic Drainage Techniques

Below are some effective lymphatic drainage massage techniques that you can incorporate into your self-care routine or seek from a trained professional.

Basic Principles of Lymphatic Drainage Massage

1. **Gentle Pressure:** Lymphatic vessels are located just beneath the skin, so gentle, light pressureis sufficient. Avoid deep or aggressive movements.
2. **Rhythmic Movements:** Use slow, rhythmic strokes to encourage the flow of lymph fluid.
3. **Direction:** Always massage towards the lymph nodes. For the upper body, this generally means moving towards the armpits and collarbone.

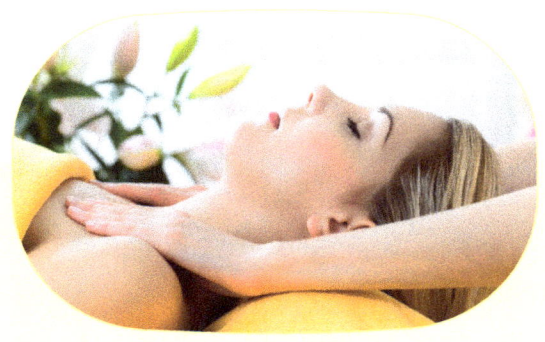

Lymphatic Massage Techniques

LYMPHATIC MASSAGES

Techniques for Lymphatic Drainage Massage

1. **Deep Breathing**

Natural deep breathing is an effective way to start your lymphatic drainage routine. It helps stimulate the flow of lymph fluid throughout the body.

- **Application:**
    - Sit or lie down in a comfortable position.
    - Take a few deep breaths in through your nose, allowing your abdomen to expand.
    - Holding your breath for a few seconds.
    - When exhaling, slowly blow out of your mouth and release your breath. Pull your abdomen in, bringing the belly button inward.
    - Keep the neck and shoulders loose and relaxed.
    - Repeat this process 5-10 times.

Lymphatic Massage Techniques

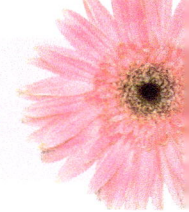

LYMPHATIC MASSAGES

Techniques for Lymphatic Drainage Massage

2. Neck Lymphatic Massage

The neck is a key area for lymphatic drainage, as many lymph nodes are located here.

- **Application**
    - Place your fingers on either side of your neck, just below your ears, and hands across each other can make it more comfortable and easier.

    - Use gentle, circular motions to massage the area for about 30 seconds.

    - Very slowly, move your fingers down towards your collarbone, first continuing the circular motions, then long, slow, light-stroking downward motions.

    - Repeat this process 5-7 times.

Lymphatic Massage Techniques

BREAST MASSAGE

BREAST SELF EXAMINATION

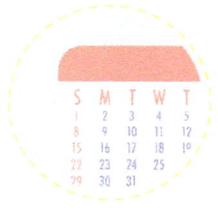

ONCE A MONTH,
2-3 DAYS AFTER PERIODS

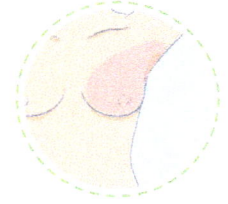

EXAMINE BREAST AND ARMPIT
WITH RAISED ARM

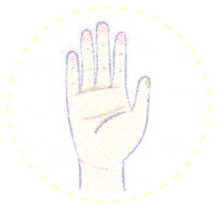

USE FINGERPADS WITH
MASSAGE OIL OR SHOWER GEL

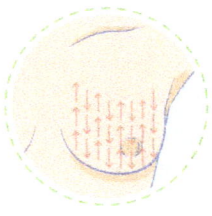

UP AND DOWN

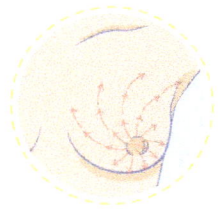

WEDGES

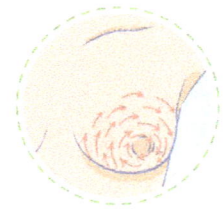

CIRCLES

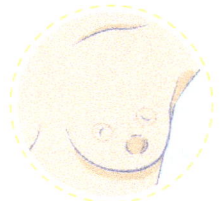

EXAMINE BREASTS IN THE MIRROR
FOR LUMPS OR SKIN DIMPLING...

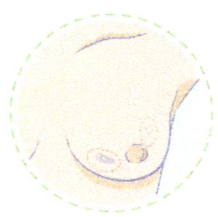

...CHANGE IN SKIN COLOR
OR TEXTURE...

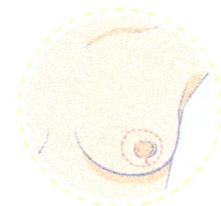

...NIPPLE DEFORMATION,
COLOR CHANGE OR LEAKS OF ANY FLUID

Lymphatic Massage Techniques

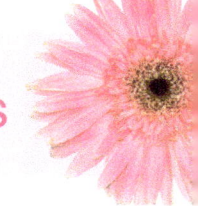

LYMPHATIC MASSAGES

Continued Techniques for Lymphatic Drainage Massage

3. **Armpit Massage**
The armpits contain numerous lymph nodes that are essential for draining lymph fluid from the upper body.

- **Application:**
  - Raise your arm and place your opposite hand under your armpit. Perform small gentle pumps to clear nodes. Make sure to keep the pumps soft and light; remember, they are located just below the skin.

  - Use gentle, circular motions to massage the armpit area for about 30 seconds.

  - Slowly move your hands down just on the side of the breast and body towards your armpit, continuing the circular motions, clearing the tissue closer to the nodes first. Then, follow with long strokes from the waist to the armpit, starting closer to the nodes and working to longer movements from your waist up to the armpit.

  - This helps the return of waste to be removed and the axillary node to remove unwanted toxins.

  - Repeat this process 5-7 times for each armpit.

Lymphatic Massage Techniques

LYMPHATIC MASSAGES

Techniques for Lymphatic Drainage Massage

4. Breast Massage
Breast massage can help promote lymphatic drainage and support the softening of the breast tissue and fluid removal.
- Application:
    - Place your fingers on the outer edge of your breast.
    - Use pads of fingers with bare skin or shower gel.
    - Finger tapping up and down the breast to feel for lumps or dense tissue.
    - Use gentle, circular motions to massage inwards towards the nipple in a wedge formation.
    - Then, perform smaller circles near the nipple to circulate the areolar area.
    - Move your fingers in a spiral pattern, covering the entire breast.
    - Continue this for about 1-2 minutes per breast.
    - Avoid applying too much pressure and focus on being gentle and rhythmic.

Lymphatic Massage Techniques

LYMPHATIC MASSAGES

5. **Abdomen Massage**

Stimulating the lymph nodes in the abdomen can help enhance lymphatic circulation, improve emotional support, and promote the movement of bowel functions.

- Application:
    - Lie on your back with your knees bent and relax the back curve.

    - Place your hands on your abdomen, just below your rib cage. To stimulate the small intestines, start with big circles and work towards smaller circles.

    - Use gentle, circular motions to massage in a clockwise direction. (Make sure you're going clockwise so you won't back up your system going in the wrong direction.)

    - Gradually move your hands down towards your lower abdomen, giving light pumps to the lower area and clearing the whole abdomen nodes.

    - Repeat this process for about 2-3 minutes.

Lymphatic Massage Techniques

LYMPHATIC MASSAGES

Tips for Effective Lymphatic Drainage Massage

- **Use Light Pressure:** The lymphatic system is close to the skin's surface, so always use gentle, light pressure when massaging to encourage fluid movement without discomfort.

- **Stay Hydrated:** Drinking plenty of water before and after the massage helps flush out toxins and supports lymphatic function.

- **Be Consistent:** Consistency is critical for best results. Perform lymphatic breast massage regularly—2-3 times a week—especially if you experience swelling or discomfort.

- **Other Practices:** Exercise, a healthy diet, and deep breathing can enhance the benefits of lymphatic drainage massage.

- **Seek Professional Help:** Consult a trained Lymphatic Drainage Therapist for more complex or severe lymphatic issues.

These simple techniques can aid in reducing swelling, promoting circulation, and enhancing breast health practices.

Chapter 6
Diet and Lifestyle

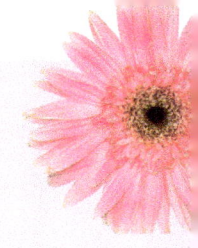

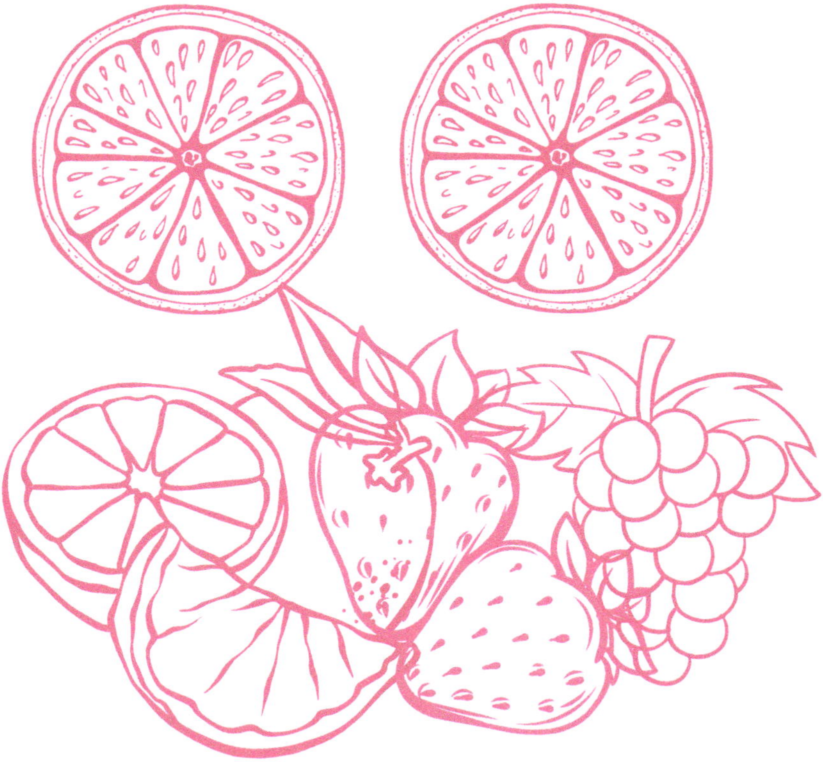

Diet and Lifestyle

Diet and Lifestyle for Optimal Breast Health

A healthy diet and lifestyle can significantly impact breast health. Nutrient-rich foods, regular exercise, and avoiding harmful substances contribute to overall well-being.

Recommendations:
- *Healthy Diet:* Include fruits, vegetables, whole grains, and lean proteins.

- *Regular Exercise:* Engage in at least 30 minutes of physical activity daily.

- *Avoid Smoking and Excessive Alcohol:* Reduce risk factors for breast diseases.

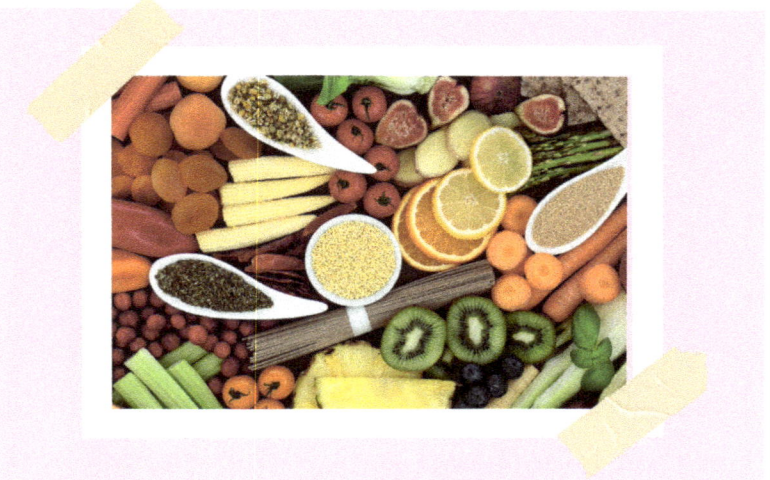

Diet and Lifestyle

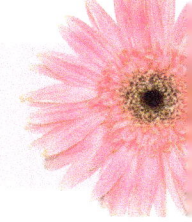

Nutrition and Diet

Certain foods can reduce inflammation, promote detoxification, and support the body's immune system.

Cruciferous Vegetables: Broccoli, kale, and cauliflower contain compounds that help detoxify the body and support breast health.

Omega-3 Fatty Acids: Found in fish, flaxseeds, and walnuts, omega-3s reduce inflammation and support healthy cell function.

Antioxidant-Rich Foods: Berries, green tea, and dark leafy greens are rich in antioxidants that protect cells from oxidative stress and may reduce the risk of breast cancer.

Flaxseeds: High in lignans, flaxseeds help balance estrogen levels, which can be essential for maintaining breast health.

Limit Processed Foods and Sugar: Reducing your intake of sugar and processed foods can decrease inflammation and the risk of hormone-related breast issues.

Diet and Lifestyle

Exercise and Movement

Regular physical activity supports lymphatic flow, reduces the risk of breast cancer, and helps maintain a healthy body weight.

- **Aerobic Exercise:** Activities like walking, running, cycling, or swimming boost circulation and improve lymphatic drainage, promoting detoxification.

- **Strength Training:** Builds muscle, supports hormonal balance, and enhances overall physical health.

- **Yoga:** Yoga improves flexibility, reduces stress, and stimulates lymphatic flow. Certain poses, like inversions and chest-opening stretches, can promote circulation and lymphatic movement in the breast area.

- **Rebounding (Mini Trampoline):** Gentle bouncing on a rebounder stimulates the lymphatic system, improving drainage and detoxification.

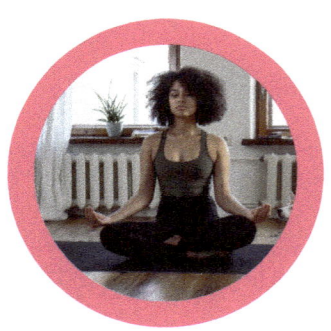

Diet and Lifestyle

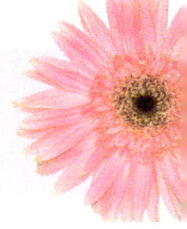

Commit to Your Health:

Staying informed and proactive can help you achieve and maintain optimal breast health. By taking these dedicated steps to support your lymphatic system, you can enhance your breast health, reduce the risk of common breast issues, and promote a sense of well-being.

Taking charge of your breast health and body is a lifelong commitment that empowers your quality of life and peace of mind. By integrating the practices discussed in this book, you invest in your breast health and full-body well-being.

Always consult with healthcare professionals and certified practitioners of traditional and holistic breast therapies for personalized advice and treatment plans.

Balanced Boobs

Key Takeaways:

1. **Understand Your Body:** Knowledge of the lymphatic system's role in breast health empowers you to make informed decisions about your care.

2. **Incorporate Lymphatic Massage:** Regular lymphatic drainage massage can help reduce swelling, improve circulation, and support detoxification.

3. **Adopt Holistic Practices:** A balanced diet, regular exercise, stress management, and natural therapies can contribute significantly to maintaining healthy breast tissue.

4. **Stay Proactive:** Regular self-examinations and professional screenings are essential for early detection and prevention of breast health issues.

5. **Seek Professional Guidance:** Always consult healthcare professionals for personalized advice and treatment plans tailored to your specific needs.

Balanced Boobs

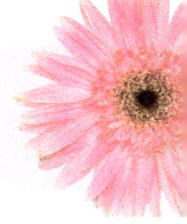

Further Resources:

For more information, support, and resources, consider reaching out to:

- American Cancer Society: www.cancer.org

- National Breast Cancer Foundation: www.nationalbreastcancer.org

- Lymphatic Education & Research Network: www.lymphaticnetwork.org

I hope that this book has provided valuable insights and practical steps to enhance lymphatic breast health. Remember, your health is in your hands, and with the proper knowledge and practices, you can achieve and maintain optimal breast health.

Balanced Boobs

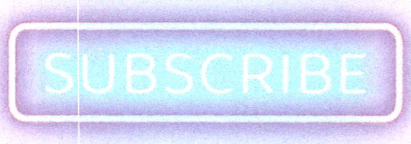

Coming soon! Please subscribe to our *Waze2Wellness* YouTube channel and Podcast. Join us weekly as we do a dive deep into alternative ways to health, wellness, and natural healing practices from a therapeutic standpoint of massage, acupuncture, herbal, and functional medicine. Each episode features interviews with health professionals and real clients providing insightful discussions along with practical tips to help you integrate these therapies into your daily life. Whether you're a wellness enthusiast or just curious about alternative healing, *Waze2Wellness* offers valuable information and inspiration to guide you on your journey to a healthier, balanced, and more vibrant life.

YT: @waze2wellness

email: waze2wellness@gmail.com

BREAST-CARE *Journal*

Date: ___/___/___

- ◯ Did self-breast exam this month?
- ◯ Have any new lumps or changes?
- ◯ Any visual size or shape changes?
- ◯ Any dimpling or redness?
- ◯ Engaged in positive thinking
- ◯ Stretching /Yoga /Meditation
- ◯ Worked out 3x or more

- ◯ Have any nipple discharge?
- ◯ Did lymphatic breast massage?
- ◯ Any pain or tenderness lately?
- ◯ Drank 6-8 glasses of water daily
- ◯ Have a clinical exam scheduled
- ◯ Ate nutrient-rich food?
- ◯ Practice health gratitude

- ◯ Annual Mammogram Scheduled

Add any additional health changes or concerns.

_____

_____

_____

_____

A LIFE OF GRATITUDE UNCLOCKS THE FULLNESS OF
A HEALTHIER MIND, BREAST AND BODY.

Breast Health Gratitude

Quietly practice a stress management of your choice & give yourself an affirmation of gratitude. Journal your experience.

A LIFE OF GRATITUDE UNCLOCKS THE FULLNESS OF
A HEALTHIER MIND, BREAST AND BODY.

BREAST-CARE *Journal*

Date: ___/___/___

- ○ Did self-breast exam this month?
- ○ Have any new lumps or changes?
- ○ Any visual size or shape changes?
- ○ Any dimpling or redness?
- ○ Engaged in positive thinking
- ○ Stretching /Yoga /Meditation
- ○ Worked out 3x or more

- ○ Have any nipple discharge?
- ○ Did lymphatic breast massage?
- ○ Any pain or tenderness lately?
- ○ Drank 6-8 glasses of water daily
- ○ Have a clinical exam scheduled
- ○ Ate nutrient-rich food?
- ○ Practice health gratitude

- ○ Annual Mammogram Scheduled

Add any additional health changes or concerns.

_____

_____

_____

_____

A LIFE OF GRATITUDE UNCLOCKS THE FULLNESS OF
A HEALTHIER MIND, BREAST AND BODY.

Breast Health Gratitude

Quietly practice a stress management of your choice & give yourself an affirmation of gratitude. Journal your experience.

A LIFE OF GRATITUDE UNCLOCKS THE FULLNESS OF
A HEALTHIER MIND, BREAST AND BODY.

BREAST-CARE *Journal*

Date: ___/___/___

- ◯ Did self-breast exam this month?
- ◯ Have any new lumps or changes?
- ◯ Any visual size or shape changes?
- ◯ Any dimpling or redness?
- ◯ Engaged in positive thinking
- ◯ Stretching /Yoga /Meditation
- ◯ Worked out 3x or more
- ◯ Have any nipple discharge?
- ◯ Did lymphatic breast massage?
- ◯ Any pain or tenderness lately?
- ◯ Drank 6-8 glasses of water daily
- ◯ Have a clinical exam scheduled
- ◯ Ate nutrient-rich food?
- ◯ Practice health gratitude
- ◯ Annual Mammogram Scheduled

Add any additional health changes or concerns.

_____

_____

_____

_____

A LIFE OF GRATITUDE UNCLOCKS THE FULLNESS OF A HEALTHIER MIND, BREAST AND BODY.

Breast Health Gratitude

Quietly practice a stress management of your choice & give yourself an affirmation of gratitude. Journal your experience.

A LIFE OF GRATITUDE UNCLOCKS THE FULLNESS OF
A HEALTHIER MIND, BREAST AND BODY.

BREAST-CARE *Journal*

Date: ___/___/___

- ◯ Did self-breast exam this month?
- ◯ Have any new lumps or changes?
- ◯ Any visual size or shape changes?
- ◯ Any dimpling or redness?
- ◯ Engaged in positive thinking
- ◯ Stretching /Yoga /Meditation
- ◯ Worked out 3x or more

- ◯ Have any nipple discharge?
- ◯ Did lymphatic breast massage?
- ◯ Any pain or tenderness lately?
- ◯ Drank 6-8 glasses of water daily
- ◯ Have a clinical exam scheduled
- ◯ Ate nutrient-rich food?
- ◯ Practice health gratitude

- ◯ Annual Mammogram Scheduled

Add any additional health changes or concerns.

_____

_____

_____

_____

A LIFE OF GRATITUDE UNCLOCKS THE FULLNESS OF
A HEALTHIER MIND, BREAST AND BODY.

Breast Health Gratitude

Quietly practice a stress management of your choice & give yourself an affirmation of gratitude. Journal your experience.

A LIFE OF GRATITUDE UNCLOCKS THE FULLNESS OF
A HEALTHIER MIND, BREAST AND BODY.

BREAST-CARE *Journal*

Date: ___/___/___

○ Did self-breast exam this month?
○ Have any new lumps or changes?
○ Any visual size or shape changes?
○ Any dimpling or redness?
○ Engaged in positive thinking
○ Stretching /Yoga /Meditation
○ Worked out 3x or more

○ Have any nipple discharge?
○ Did lymphatic breast massage?
○ Any pain or tenderness lately?
○ Drank 6-8 glasses of water daily
○ Have a clinical exam scheduled
○ Ate nutrient-rich food?
○ Practice health gratitude

○ Annual Mammogram Scheduled

Add any additional health changes or concerns.

___

A LIFE OF GRATITUDE UNCLOCKS THE FULLNESS OF A HEALTHIER MIND, BREAST AND BODY.

Breast Health Gratitude

Quietly practice a stress management of your choice & give yourself an affirmation of gratitude. Journal your experience.

A LIFE OF GRATITUDE UNCLOCKS THE FULLNESS OF
A HEALTHIER MIND, BREAST AND BODY.

BREAST-CARE *Journal*

Date: ___/___/___

- ○ Did self-breast exam this month?
- ○ Have any new lumps or changes?
- ○ Any visual size or shape changes?
- ○ Any dimpling or redness?
- ○ Engaged in positive thinking
- ○ Stretching /Yoga /Meditation
- ○ Worked out 3x or more

- ○ Have any nipple discharge?
- ○ Did lymphatic breast massage?
- ○ Any pain or tenderness lately?
- ○ Drank 6-8 glasses of water daily
- ○ Have a clinical exam scheduled
- ○ Ate nutrient-rich food?
- ○ Practice health gratitude

- ○ Annual Mammogram Scheduled

Add any additional health changes or concerns.

_____

_____

_____

_____

A LIFE OF GRATITUDE UNCLOCKS THE FULLNESS OF
A HEALTHIER MIND, BREAST AND BODY.

Breast Health Gratitude

Quietly practice a stress management of your choice & give yourself an affirmation of gratitude. Journal your experience.

A LIFE OF GRATITUDE UNCLOCKS THE FULLNESS OF
A HEALTHIER MIND, BREAST AND BODY.

BREAST-CARE *Journal*

Date: ___/___/___

- ○ Did self-breast exam this month?
- ○ Have any new lumps or changes?
- ○ Any visual size or shape changes?
- ○ Any dimpling or redness?
- ○ Engaged in positive thinking
- ○ Stretching /Yoga /Meditation
- ○ Worked out 3x or more

- ○ Have any nipple discharge?
- ○ Did lymphatic breast massage?
- ○ Any pain or tenderness lately?
- ○ Drank 6-8 glasses of water daily
- ○ Have a clinical exam scheduled
- ○ Ate nutrient-rich food?
- ○ Practice health gratitude

- ○ Annual Mammogram Scheduled

Add any additional health changes or concerns.

_____
_____
_____
_____

A LIFE OF GRATITUDE UNCLOCKS THE FULLNESS OF
A HEALTHIER MIND, BREAST AND BODY.

Breast Health Gratitude

Quietly practice a stress management of your choice & give yourself an affirmation of gratitude. Journal your experience.

A LIFE OF GRATITUDE UNCLOCKS THE FULLNESS OF
A HEALTHIER MIND, BREAST AND BODY.

BREAST-CARE *Journal*

Date: ___/___/___

○ Did self-breast exam this month?
○ Have any new lumps or changes?
○ Any visual size or shape changes?
○ Any dimpling or redness?
○ Engaged in positive thinking
○ Stretching /Yoga /Meditation
○ Worked out 3x or more

○ Have any nipple discharge?
○ Did lymphatic breast massage?
○ Any pain or tenderness lately?
○ Drank 6-8 glasses of water daily
○ Have a clinical exam scheduled
○ Ate nutrient-rich food?
○ Practice health gratitude

○ Annual Mammogram Scheduled

Add any additional health changes or concerns.

_____
_____
_____
_____

A LIFE OF GRATITUDE UNCLOCKS THE FULLNESS OF A HEALTHIER MIND, BREAST AND BODY.

Breast Health Gratitude

Quietly practice a stress management of your choice & give yourself an affirmation of gratitude. Journal your experience.

A LIFE OF GRATITUDE UNCLOCKS THE FULLNESS OF
A HEALTHIER MIND, BREAST AND BODY.

BREAST-CARE *Journal*

Date: ___/___/___

- ○ Did self-breast exam this month?
- ○ Have any new lumps or changes?
- ○ Any visual size or shape changes?
- ○ Any dimpling or redness?
- ○ Engaged in positive thinking
- ○ Stretching / Yoga / Meditation
- ○ Worked out 3x or more
- ○ Have any nipple discharge?
- ○ Did lymphatic breast massage?
- ○ Any pain or tenderness lately?
- ○ Drank 6-8 glasses of water daily
- ○ Have a clinical exam scheduled
- ○ Ate nutrient-rich food?
- ○ Practice health gratitude
- ○ Annual Mammogram Scheduled

Add any additional health changes or concerns.

_____

_____

_____

_____

A LIFE OF GRATITUDE UNCLOCKS THE FULLNESS OF A HEALTHIER MIND, BREAST AND BODY.

Breast Health Gratitude

Quietly practice a stress management of your choice & give yourself an affirmation of gratitude. Journal your experience.

A LIFE OF GRATITUDE UNCLOCKS THE FULLNESS OF
A HEALTHIER MIND, BREAST AND BODY.

BREAST-CARE *Journal*

Date: ___/___/___

- ◯ Did self-breast exam this month?
- ◯ Have any new lumps or changes?
- ◯ Any visual size or shape changes?
- ◯ Any dimpling or redness?
- ◯ Engaged in positive thinking
- ◯ Stretching /Yoga /Meditation
- ◯ Worked out 3x or more

- ◯ Have any nipple discharge?
- ◯ Did lymphatic breast massage?
- ◯ Any pain or tenderness lately?
- ◯ Drank 6-8 glasses of water daily
- ◯ Have a clinical exam scheduled
- ◯ Ate nutrient-rich food?
- ◯ Practice health gratitude

- ◯ Annual Mammogram Scheduled

Add any additional health changes or concerns.

___

___

___

___

A LIFE OF GRATITUDE UNCLOCKS THE FULLNESS OF A HEALTHIER MIND, BREAST AND BODY.

Breast Health Gratitude

Quietly practice a stress management of your choice & give yourself an affirmation of gratitude. Journal your experience.

A LIFE OF GRATITUDE UNCLOCKS THE FULLNESS OF
A HEALTHIER MIND, BREAST AND BODY.

BREAST-CARE *Journal*

Date: ___/___/___

- ○ Did self-breast exam this month?
- ○ Have any new lumps or changes?
- ○ Any visual size or shape changes?
- ○ Any dimpling or redness?
- ○ Engaged in positive thinking
- ○ Stretching /Yoga /Meditation
- ○ Worked out 3x or more

- ○ Have any nipple discharge?
- ○ Did lymphatic breast massage?
- ○ Any pain or tenderness lately?
- ○ Drank 6-8 glasses of water daily
- ○ Have a clinical exam scheduled
- ○ Ate nutrient-rich food?
- ○ Practice health gratitude

- ○ Annual Mammogram Scheduled

Add any additional health changes or concerns.

___

A LIFE OF GRATITUDE UNCLOCKS THE FULLNESS OF
A HEALTHIER MIND, BREAST AND BODY.

Breast Health Gratitude

Quietly practice a stress management of your choice & give yourself an affirmation of gratitude. Journal your experience.

A LIFE OF GRATITUDE UNCLOCKS THE FULLNESS OF
A HEALTHIER MIND, BREAST AND BODY.

BREAST-CARE *Journal*

Date: ___/___/___

- ◯ Did self-breast exam this month?
- ◯ Have any new lumps or changes?
- ◯ Any visual size or shape changes?
- ◯ Any dimpling or redness?
- ◯ Engaged in positive thinking
- ◯ Stretching /Yoga /Meditation
- ◯ Worked out 3x or more

- ◯ Have any nipple discharge?
- ◯ Did lymphatic breast massage?
- ◯ Any pain or tenderness lately?
- ◯ Drank 6-8 glasses of water daily
- ◯ Have a clinical exam scheduled
- ◯ Ate nutrient-rich food?
- ◯ Practice health gratitude

- ◯ Annual Mammogram Scheduled

Add any additional health changes or concerns.

_____

_____

_____

_____

A LIFE OF GRATITUDE UNCLOCKS THE FULLNESS OF A HEALTHIER MIND, BREAST AND BODY.

Breast Health Gratitude

Quietly practice a stress management of your choice & give yourself an affirmation of gratitude. Journal your experience.

A LIFE OF GRATITUDE UNCLOCKS THE FULLNESS OF
A HEALTHIER MIND, BREAST AND BODY.

BREAST-CARE *Journal*

Date: ___/___/___

- ○ Did self-breast exam this month?
- ○ Have any new lumps or changes?
- ○ Any visual size or shape changes?
- ○ Any dimpling or redness?
- ○ Engaged in positive thinking
- ○ Stretching /Yoga /Meditation
- ○ Worked out 3x or more

- ○ Have any nipple discharge?
- ○ Did lymphatic breast massage?
- ○ Any pain or tenderness lately?
- ○ Drank 6-8 glasses of water daily
- ○ Have a clinical exam scheduled
- ○ Ate nutrient-rich food?
- ○ Practice health gratitude

- ○ Annual Mammogram Scheduled

Add any additional health changes or concerns.

_____

_____

_____

_____

A LIFE OF GRATITUDE UNCLOCKS THE FULLNESS OF
A HEALTHIER MIND, BREAST AND BODY.

Breast Health Gratitude

Quietly practice a stress management of your choice & give yourself an affirmation of gratitude. Journal your experience.

A LIFE OF GRATITUDE UNCLOCKS THE FULLNESS OF
A HEALTHIER MIND, BREAST AND BODY.

BREAST-CARE *Journal*

Date: ___ / ___ / ___

- ○ Did self-breast exam this month?
- ○ Have any new lumps or changes?
- ○ Any visual size or shape changes?
- ○ Any dimpling or redness?
- ○ Engaged in positive thinking
- ○ Stretching / Yoga / Meditation
- ○ Worked out 3x or more

- ○ Have any nipple discharge?
- ○ Did lymphatic breast massage?
- ○ Any pain or tenderness lately?
- ○ Drank 6-8 glasses of water daily
- ○ Have a clinical exam scheduled
- ○ Ate nutrient-rich food?
- ○ Practice health gratitude

- ○ Annual Mammogram Scheduled

Add any additional health changes or concerns.

_____

_____

_____

_____

A LIFE OF GRATITUDE UNCLOCKS THE FULLNESS OF
A HEALTHIER MIND, BREAST AND BODY.

Breast Health Gratitude

Quietly practice a stress management of your choice & give yourself an affirmation of gratitude. Journal your experience.

A LIFE OF GRATITUDE UNCLOCKS THE FULLNESS OF
A HEALTHIER MIND, BREAST AND BODY.

BREAST-CARE *Journal*

Date: ___/___/___

- ◯ Did self-breast exam this month?
- ◯ Have any new lumps or changes?
- ◯ Any visual size or shape changes?
- ◯ Any dimpling or redness?
- ◯ Engaged in positive thinking
- ◯ Stretching /Yoga /Meditation
- ◯ Worked out 3x or more

- ◯ Have any nipple discharge?
- ◯ Did lymphatic breast massage?
- ◯ Any pain or tenderness lately?
- ◯ Drank 6-8 glasses of water daily
- ◯ Have a clinical exam scheduled
- ◯ Ate nutrient-rich food?
- ◯ Practice health gratitude

- ◯ Annual Mammogram Scheduled

Add any additional health changes or concerns.

_____

_____

_____

_____

A LIFE OF GRATITUDE UNCLOCKS THE FULLNESS OF A HEALTHIER MIND, BREAST AND BODY.

Breast Health Gratitude

Quietly practice a stress management of your choice & give yourself an affirmation of gratitude. Journal your experience.

_____

_____

_____

_____

_____

_____

_____

_____

_____

_____

_____

_____

A LIFE OF GRATITUDE UNCLOCKS THE FULLNESS OF A HEALTHIER MIND, BREAST AND BODY.

BREAST-CARE *Journal*

Date: ___/___/___

- ◯ Did self-breast exam this month?
- ◯ Have any new lumps or changes?
- ◯ Any visual size or shape changes?
- ◯ Any dimpling or redness?
- ◯ Engaged in positive thinking
- ◯ Stretching /Yoga /Meditation
- ◯ Worked out 3x or more

- ◯ Have any nipple discharge?
- ◯ Did lymphatic breast massage?
- ◯ Any pain or tenderness lately?
- ◯ Drank 6-8 glasses of water daily
- ◯ Have a clinical exam scheduled
- ◯ Ate nutrient-rich food?
- ◯ Practice health gratitude

- ◯ Annual Mammogram Scheduled

Add any additional health changes or concerns.

_____

_____

_____

A LIFE OF GRATITUDE UNCLOCKS THE FULLNESS OF
A HEALTHIER MIND, BREAST AND BODY.

Breast Health Gratitude

Quietly practice a stress management of your choice & give yourself an affirmation of gratitude. Journal your experience.

A LIFE OF GRATITUDE UNCLOCKS THE FULLNESS OF
A HEALTHIER MIND, BREAST AND BODY.

BREAST-CARE *Journal*

Date: ___/___/___

○ Did self-breast exam this month?
○ Have any new lumps or changes?
○ Any visual size or shape changes?
○ Any dimpling or redness?
○ Engaged in positive thinking
○ Stretching /Yoga /Meditation
○ Worked out 3x or more

○ Have any nipple discharge?
○ Did lymphatic breast massage?
○ Any pain or tenderness lately?
○ Drank 6-8 glasses of water daily
○ Have a clinical exam scheduled
○ Ate nutrient-rich food?
○ Practice health gratitude

○ Annual Mammogram Scheduled

Add any additional health changes or concerns.

_____
_____
_____
_____

A LIFE OF GRATITUDE UNCLOCKS THE FULLNESS OF
A HEALTHIER MIND, BREAST AND BODY.

Breast Health Gratitude

Quietly practice a stress management of your choice & give yourself an affirmation of gratitude. Journal your experience.

A LIFE OF GRATITUDE UNCLOCKS THE FULLNESS OF
A HEALTHIER MIND, BREAST AND BODY.

BREAST-CARE *Journal*

Date: ___/___/___

- ◯ Did self-breast exam this month?
- ◯ Have any new lumps or changes?
- ◯ Any visual size or shape changes?
- ◯ Any dimpling or redness?
- ◯ Engaged in positive thinking
- ◯ Stretching /Yoga /Meditation
- ◯ Worked out 3x or more

- ◯ Have any nipple discharge?
- ◯ Did lymphatic breast massage?
- ◯ Any pain or tenderness lately?
- ◯ Drank 6-8 glasses of water daily
- ◯ Have a clinical exam scheduled
- ◯ Ate nutrient-rich food?
- ◯ Practice health gratitude

- ◯ Annual Mammogram Scheduled

Add any additional health changes or concerns.

_____

_____

_____

_____

A LIFE OF GRATITUDE UNCLOCKS THE FULLNESS OF
A HEALTHIER MIND, BREAST AND BODY.

Breast Health Gratitude

Quietly practice a stress management of your choice & give yourself an affirmation of gratitude. Journal your experience.

A LIFE OF GRATITUDE UNCLOCKS THE FULLNESS OF
A HEALTHIER MIND, BREAST AND BODY.

BREAST-CARE *Journal*

Date: ___ / ___ / ___

- ◯ Did self-breast exam this month?
- ◯ Have any new lumps or changes?
- ◯ Any visual size or shape changes?
- ◯ Any dimpling or redness?
- ◯ Engaged in positive thinking
- ◯ Stretching / Yoga / Meditation
- ◯ Worked out 3x or more

- ◯ Have any nipple discharge?
- ◯ Did lymphatic breast massage?
- ◯ Any pain or tenderness lately?
- ◯ Drank 6-8 glasses of water daily
- ◯ Have a clinical exam scheduled
- ◯ Ate nutrient-rich food?
- ◯ Practice health gratitude

- ◯ Annual Mammogram Scheduled

Add any additional health changes or concerns.

A LIFE OF GRATITUDE UNCLOCKS THE FULLNESS OF A HEALTHIER MIND, BREAST AND BODY.

Breast Health Gratitude

Quietly practice a stress management of your choice & give yourself an affirmation of gratitude. Journal your experience.

A LIFE OF GRATITUDE UNCLOCKS THE FULLNESS OF
A HEALTHIER MIND, BREAST AND BODY.

BREAST-CARE *Journal*

Date: ___/___/___

- ○ Did self-breast exam this month?
- ○ Have any new lumps or changes?
- ○ Any visual size or shape changes?
- ○ Any dimpling or redness?
- ○ Engaged in positive thinking
- ○ Stretching /Yoga /Meditation
- ○ Worked out 3x or more

- ○ Have any nipple discharge?
- ○ Did lymphatic breast massage?
- ○ Any pain or tenderness lately?
- ○ Drank 6-8 glasses of water daily
- ○ Have a clinical exam scheduled
- ○ Ate nutrient-rich food?
- ○ Practice health gratitude

- ○ Annual Mammogram Scheduled

Add any additional health changes or concerns.

_____

_____

_____

_____

A LIFE OF GRATITUDE UNCLOCKS THE FULLNESS OF
A HEALTHIER MIND, BREAST AND BODY.

Breast Health Gratitude

Quietly practice a stress management of your choice & give yourself an affirmation of gratitude. Journal your experience.

A LIFE OF GRATITUDE UNCLOCKS THE FULLNESS OF
A HEALTHIER MIND, BREAST AND BODY.

BREAST-CARE *Journal*

Date: ___/___/___

- ◯ Did self-breast exam this month?
- ◯ Have any new lumps or changes?
- ◯ Any visual size or shape changes?
- ◯ Any dimpling or redness?
- ◯ Engaged in positive thinking
- ◯ Stretching /Yoga /Meditation
- ◯ Worked out 3x or more

- ◯ Have any nipple discharge?
- ◯ Did lymphatic breast massage?
- ◯ Any pain or tenderness lately?
- ◯ Drank 6-8 glasses of water daily
- ◯ Have a clinical exam scheduled
- ◯ Ate nutrient-rich food?
- ◯ Practice health gratitude

- ◯ Annual Mammogram Scheduled

Add any additional health changes or concerns.

A LIFE OF GRATITUDE UNCLOCKS THE FULLNESS OF
A HEALTHIER MIND, BREAST AND BODY.

Breast Health Gratitude

Quietly practice a stress management of your choice & give yourself an affirmation of gratitude. Journal your experience.

A LIFE OF GRATITUDE UNCLOCKS THE FULLNESS OF
A HEALTHIER MIND, BREAST AND BODY.

BREAST-CARE *Journal*

Date: ___/___/___

- ◯ Did self-breast exam this month?
- ◯ Have any new lumps or changes?
- ◯ Any visual size or shape changes?
- ◯ Any dimpling or redness?
- ◯ Engaged in positive thinking
- ◯ Stretching /Yoga /Meditation
- ◯ Worked out 3x or more

- ◯ Have any nipple discharge?
- ◯ Did lymphatic breast massage?
- ◯ Any pain or tenderness lately?
- ◯ Drank 6-8 glasses of water daily
- ◯ Have a clinical exam scheduled
- ◯ Ate nutrient-rich food?
- ◯ Practice health gratitude

- ◯ Annual Mammogram Scheduled

Add any additional health changes or concerns.

_____
_____
_____
_____

A LIFE OF GRATITUDE UNCLOCKS THE FULLNESS OF A HEALTHIER MIND, BREAST AND BODY.

Breast Health Gratitude

Quietly practice a stress management of your choice & give yourself an affirmation of gratitude. Journal your experience.

A LIFE OF GRATITUDE UNCLOCKS THE FULLNESS OF
A HEALTHIER MIND, BREAST AND BODY.

BREAST-CARE *Journal*

Date: ___ / ___ / ___

- ◯ Did self-breast exam this month?
- ◯ Have any new lumps or changes?
- ◯ Any visual size or shape changes?
- ◯ Any dimpling or redness?
- ◯ Engaged in positive thinking
- ◯ Stretching / Yoga / Meditation
- ◯ Worked out 3x or more

- ◯ Have any nipple discharge?
- ◯ Did lymphatic breast massage?
- ◯ Any pain or tenderness lately?
- ◯ Drank 6-8 glasses of water daily
- ◯ Have a clinical exam scheduled
- ◯ Ate nutrient-rich food?
- ◯ Practice health gratitude

- ◯ Annual Mammogram Scheduled

Add any additional health changes or concerns.

___

A LIFE OF GRATITUDE UNCLOCKS THE FULLNESS OF A HEALTHIER MIND, BREAST AND BODY.

Breast Health Gratitude

Quietly practice a stress management of your choice & give yourself an affirmation of gratitude. Journal your experience.

A LIFE OF GRATITUDE UNCLOCKS THE FULLNESS OF
A HEALTHIER MIND, BREAST AND BODY.

BREAST-CARE *Journal*

Date: ___/___/___

- ☐ Did self-breast exam this month?
- ☐ Have any new lumps or changes?
- ☐ Any visual size or shape changes?
- ☐ Any dimpling or redness?
- ☐ Engaged in positive thinking
- ☐ Stretching /Yoga /Meditation
- ☐ Worked out 3x or more

- ☐ Have any nipple discharge?
- ☐ Did lymphatic breast massage?
- ☐ Any pain or tenderness lately?
- ☐ Drank 6-8 glasses of water daily
- ☐ Have a clinical exam scheduled
- ☐ Ate nutrient-rich food?
- ☐ Practice health gratitude

- ☐ Annual Mammogram Scheduled

Add any additional health changes or concerns.

_____

_____

_____

A LIFE OF GRATITUDE UNCLOCKS THE FULLNESS OF
A HEALTHIER MIND, BREAST AND BODY.

Breast Health Gratitude

Quietly practice a stress management of your choice & give yourself an affirmation of gratitude. Journal your experience.

A LIFE OF GRATITUDE UNCLOCKS THE FULLNESS OF
A HEALTHIER MIND, BREAST AND BODY.

BREAST-CARE *Journal*

Date: ___/___/___

○ Did self-breast exam this month?
○ Have any new lumps or changes?
○ Any visual size or shape changes?
○ Any dimpling or redness?
○ Engaged in positive thinking
○ Stretching /Yoga /Meditation
○ Worked out 3x or more

○ Have any nipple discharge?
○ Did lymphatic breast massage?
○ Any pain or tenderness lately?
○ Drank 6-8 glasses of water daily
○ Have a clinical exam scheduled
○ Ate nutrient-rich food?
○ Practice health gratitude

○ Annual Mammogram Scheduled

Add any additional health changes or concerns.

A LIFE OF GRATITUDE UNCLOCKS THE FULLNESS OF
A HEALTHIER MIND, BREAST AND BODY.

Breast Health Gratitude

Quietly practice a stress management of your choice & give yourself an affirmation of gratitude. Journal your experience.

_____

_____

_____

_____

_____

_____

_____

_____

_____

_____

_____

_____

_____

_____

A LIFE OF GRATITUDE UNCLOCKS THE FULLNESS OF
A HEALTHIER MIND, BREAST AND BODY.

BREAST-CARE *Journal*

Date: ___ / ___ / ___

- ○ Did self-breast exam this month?
- ○ Have any new lumps or changes?
- ○ Any visual size or shape changes?
- ○ Any dimpling or redness?
- ○ Engaged in positive thinking
- ○ Stretching / Yoga / Meditation
- ○ Worked out 3x or more

- ○ Have any nipple discharge?
- ○ Did lymphatic breast massage?
- ○ Any pain or tenderness lately?
- ○ Drank 6-8 glasses of water daily
- ○ Have a clinical exam scheduled
- ○ Ate nutrient-rich food?
- ○ Practice health gratitude

- ○ Annual Mammogram Scheduled

Add any additional health changes or concerns.

_____

_____

_____

_____

A LIFE OF GRATITUDE UNCLOCKS THE FULLNESS OF A HEALTHIER MIND, BREAST AND BODY.

Breast Health Gratitude

Quietly practice a stress management of your choice & give yourself an affirmation of gratitude. Journal your experience.

A LIFE OF GRATITUDE UNCLOCKS THE FULLNESS OF
A HEALTHIER MIND, BREAST AND BODY.

BREAST-CARE *Journal*

Date: ___/___/___

- ◯ Did self-breast exam this month?
- ◯ Have any new lumps or changes?
- ◯ Any visual size or shape changes?
- ◯ Any dimpling or redness?
- ◯ Engaged in positive thinking
- ◯ Stretching /Yoga /Meditation
- ◯ Worked out 3x or more

- ◯ Have any nipple discharge?
- ◯ Did lymphatic breast massage?
- ◯ Any pain or tenderness lately?
- ◯ Drank 6-8 glasses of water daily
- ◯ Have a clinical exam scheduled
- ◯ Ate nutrient-rich food?
- ◯ Practice health gratitude

- ◯ Annual Mammogram Scheduled

Add any additional health changes or concerns.

_____
_____
_____
_____

A LIFE OF GRATITUDE UNCLOCKS THE FULLNESS OF A HEALTHIER MIND, BREAST AND BODY.

Breast Health Gratitude

Quietly practice a stress management of your choice & give yourself an affirmation of gratitude. Journal your experience.

A LIFE OF GRATITUDE UNCLOCKS THE FULLNESS OF
A HEALTHIER MIND, BREAST AND BODY.

BREAST-CARE *Journal*

Date: ___/___/___

- ◯ Did self-breast exam this month?
- ◯ Have any new lumps or changes?
- ◯ Any visual size or shape changes?
- ◯ Any dimpling or redness?
- ◯ Engaged in positive thinking
- ◯ Stretching /Yoga /Meditation
- ◯ Worked out 3x or more

- ◯ Have any nipple discharge?
- ◯ Did lymphatic breast massage?
- ◯ Any pain or tenderness lately?
- ◯ Drank 6-8 glasses of water daily
- ◯ Have a clinical exam scheduled
- ◯ Ate nutrient-rich food?
- ◯ Practice health gratitude

- ◯ Annual Mammogram Scheduled

Add any additional health changes or concerns.

_____

_____

_____

A LIFE OF GRATITUDE UNCLOCKS THE FULLNESS OF A HEALTHIER MIND, BREAST AND BODY.

Breast Health Gratitude

Quietly practice a stress management of your choice & give yourself an affirmation of gratitude. Journal your experience.

A LIFE OF GRATITUDE UNCLOCKS THE FULLNESS OF
A HEALTHIER MIND, BREAST AND BODY.

BREAST-CARE *Journal*

Date: ___/___/___

- ○ Did self-breast exam this month?
- ○ Have any new lumps or changes?
- ○ Any visual size or shape changes?
- ○ Any dimpling or redness?
- ○ Engaged in positive thinking
- ○ Stretching /Yoga /Meditation
- ○ Worked out 3x or more

- ○ Have any nipple discharge?
- ○ Did lymphatic breast massage?
- ○ Any pain or tenderness lately?
- ○ Drank 6-8 glasses of water daily
- ○ Have a clinical exam scheduled
- ○ Ate nutrient-rich food?
- ○ Practice health gratitude

- ○ Annual Mammogram Scheduled

Add any additional health changes or concerns.

_____

_____

_____

_____

A LIFE OF GRATITUDE UNCLOCKS THE FULLNESS OF
A HEALTHIER MIND, BREAST AND BODY.

Breast Health Gratitude

Quietly practice a stress management of your choice & give yourself an affirmation of gratitude. Journal your experience.

A LIFE OF GRATITUDE UNCLOCKS THE FULLNESS OF
A HEALTHIER MIND, BREAST AND BODY.

BREAST-CARE *Journal*

Date: ___/___/___

- ◯ Did self-breast exam this month?
- ◯ Have any new lumps or changes?
- ◯ Any visual size or shape changes?
- ◯ Any dimpling or redness?
- ◯ Engaged in positive thinking
- ◯ Stretching /Yoga /Meditation
- ◯ Worked out 3x or more

- ◯ Have any nipple discharge?
- ◯ Did lymphatic breast massage?
- ◯ Any pain or tenderness lately?
- ◯ Drank 6-8 glasses of water daily
- ◯ Have a clinical exam scheduled
- ◯ Ate nutrient-rich food?
- ◯ Practice health gratitude

- ◯ Annual Mammogram Scheduled

Add any additional health changes or concerns.

_____

_____

_____

_____

A LIFE OF GRATITUDE UNCLOCKS THE FULLNESS OF A HEALTHIER MIND, BREAST AND BODY.

Breast Health Gratitude

Quietly practice a stress management of your choice & give yourself an affirmation of gratitude. Journal your experience.

A LIFE OF GRATITUDE UNCLOCKS THE FULLNESS OF
A HEALTHIER MIND, BREAST AND BODY.

BREAST-CARE *Journal*

Date: ___/___/___

- ◯ Did self-breast exam this month?
- ◯ Have any new lumps or changes?
- ◯ Any visual size or shape changes?
- ◯ Any dimpling or redness?
- ◯ Engaged in positive thinking
- ◯ Stretching /Yoga /Meditation
- ◯ Worked out 3x or more

- ◯ Have any nipple discharge?
- ◯ Did lymphatic breast massage?
- ◯ Any pain or tenderness lately?
- ◯ Drank 6-8 glasses of water daily
- ◯ Have a clinical exam scheduled
- ◯ Ate nutrient-rich food?
- ◯ Practice health gratitude

- ◯ Annual Mammogram Scheduled

Add any additional health changes or concerns.

___

A LIFE OF GRATITUDE UNCLOCKS THE FULLNESS OF A HEALTHIER MIND, BREAST AND BODY.

Breast Health Gratitude

Quietly practice a stress management of your choice & give yourself an affirmation of gratitude. Journal your experience.

A LIFE OF GRATITUDE UNCLOCKS THE FULLNESS OF
A HEALTHIER MIND, BREAST AND BODY.

BREAST-CARE *Journal*

Date: ___/___/___

○ Did self-breast exam this month?
○ Have any new lumps or changes?
○ Any visual size or shape changes?
○ Any dimpling or redness?
○ Engaged in positive thinking
○ Stretching /Yoga /Meditation
○ Worked out 3x or more

○ Have any nipple discharge?
○ Did lymphatic breast massage?
○ Any pain or tenderness lately?
○ Drank 6-8 glasses of water daily
○ Have a clinical exam scheduled
○ Ate nutrient-rich food?
○ Practice health gratitude

○ Annual Mammogram Scheduled

Add any additional health changes or concerns.

_____
_____
_____
_____

A LIFE OF GRATITUDE UNCLOCKS THE FULLNESS OF
A HEALTHIER MIND, BREAST AND BODY.

Breast Health Gratitude

Quietly practice a stress management of your choice & give yourself an affirmation of gratitude. Journal your experience.

A LIFE OF GRATITUDE UNCLOCKS THE FULLNESS OF
A HEALTHIER MIND, BREAST AND BODY.

BREAST-CARE *Journal*

Date: ___/___/___

○ Did self-breast exam this month?
○ Have any new lumps or changes?
○ Any visual size or shape changes?
○ Any dimpling or redness?
○ Engaged in positive thinking
○ Stretching /Yoga /Meditation
○ Worked out 3x or more

○ Have any nipple discharge?
○ Did lymphatic breast massage?
○ Any pain or tenderness lately?
○ Drank 6-8 glasses of water daily
○ Have a clinical exam scheduled
○ Ate nutrient-rich food?
○ Practice health gratitude

○ Annual Mammogram Scheduled

Add any additional health changes or concerns.

A LIFE OF GRATITUDE UNCLOCKS THE FULLNESS OF
A HEALTHIER MIND, BREAST AND BODY.

Breast Health Gratitude

Quietly practice a stress management of your choice & give yourself an affirmation of gratitude. Journal your experience.

A LIFE OF GRATITUDE UNCLOCKS THE FULLNESS OF
A HEALTHIER MIND, BREAST AND BODY.

BREAST-CARE *Journal*

Date: ___/___/___

- ○ Did self-breast exam this month?
- ○ Have any new lumps or changes?
- ○ Any visual size or shape changes?
- ○ Any dimpling or redness?
- ○ Engaged in positive thinking
- ○ Stretching /Yoga /Meditation
- ○ Worked out 3x or more

- ○ Have any nipple discharge?
- ○ Did lymphatic breast massage?
- ○ Any pain or tenderness lately?
- ○ Drank 6-8 glasses of water daily
- ○ Have a clinical exam scheduled
- ○ Ate nutrient-rich food?
- ○ Practice health gratitude

- ○ Annual Mammogram Scheduled

Add any additional health changes or concerns.

_____

_____

_____

_____

A LIFE OF GRATITUDE UNCLOCKS THE FULLNESS OF A HEALTHIER MIND, BREAST AND BODY.

Breast Health Gratitude

Quietly practice a stress management of your choice & give yourself an affirmation of gratitude. Journal your experience.

A LIFE OF GRATITUDE UNCLOCKS THE FULLNESS OF
A HEALTHIER MIND, BREAST AND BODY.

BREAST-CARE *Journal*

Date: ___ / ___ / ___

- ◯ Did self-breast exam this month?
- ◯ Have any new lumps or changes?
- ◯ Any visual size or shape changes?
- ◯ Any dimpling or redness?
- ◯ Engaged in positive thinking
- ◯ Stretching / Yoga / Meditation
- ◯ Worked out 3x or more

- ◯ Have any nipple discharge?
- ◯ Did lymphatic breast massage?
- ◯ Any pain or tenderness lately?
- ◯ Drank 6-8 glasses of water daily
- ◯ Have a clinical exam scheduled
- ◯ Ate nutrient-rich food?
- ◯ Practice health gratitude

- ◯ Annual Mammogram Scheduled

Add any additional health changes or concerns.

_____

_____

_____

_____

A LIFE OF GRATITUDE UNCLOCKS THE FULLNESS OF
A HEALTHIER MIND, BREAST AND BODY.

Breast Health Gratitude

Quietly practice a stress management of your choice & give yourself an affirmation of gratitude. Journal your experience.

A LIFE OF GRATITUDE UNCLOCKS THE FULLNESS OF
A HEALTHIER MIND, BREAST AND BODY.

BREAST-CARE *Journal*

Date: ___/___/___

- ○ Did self-breast exam this month?
- ○ Have any new lumps or changes?
- ○ Any visual size or shape changes?
- ○ Any dimpling or redness?
- ○ Engaged in positive thinking
- ○ Stretching /Yoga /Meditation
- ○ Worked out 3x or more

- ○ Have any nipple discharge?
- ○ Did lymphatic breast massage?
- ○ Any pain or tenderness lately?
- ○ Drank 6-8 glasses of water daily
- ○ Have a clinical exam scheduled
- ○ Ate nutrient-rich food?
- ○ Practice health gratitude

- ○ Annual Mammogram Scheduled

Add any additional health changes or concerns.

A LIFE OF GRATITUDE UNCLOCKS THE FULLNESS OF A HEALTHIER MIND, BREAST AND BODY.

Breast Health Gratitude

Quietly practice a stress management of your choice & give yourself an affirmation of gratitude. Journal your experience.

A LIFE OF GRATITUDE UNCLOCKS THE FULLNESS OF
A HEALTHIER MIND, BREAST AND BODY.

BREAST-CARE *Journal*

Date: ___ / ___ / ___

- ○ Did self-breast exam this month?
- ○ Have any new lumps or changes?
- ○ Any visual size or shape changes?
- ○ Any dimpling or redness?
- ○ Engaged in positive thinking
- ○ Stretching / Yoga / Meditation
- ○ Worked out 3x or more

- ○ Have any nipple discharge?
- ○ Did lymphatic breast massage?
- ○ Any pain or tenderness lately?
- ○ Drank 6-8 glasses of water daily
- ○ Have a clinical exam scheduled
- ○ Ate nutrient-rich food?
- ○ Practice health gratitude

- ○ Annual Mammogram Scheduled

Add any additional health changes or concerns.

_____

_____

_____

_____

A LIFE OF GRATITUDE UNCLOCKS THE FULLNESS OF
A HEALTHIER MIND, BREAST AND BODY.

Breast Health Gratitude

Quietly practice a stress management of your choice & give yourself an affirmation of gratitude. Journal your experience.

_____

_____

_____

_____

_____

_____

_____

_____

_____

_____

_____

_____

_____

A LIFE OF GRATITUDE UNCLOCKS THE FULLNESS OF
A HEALTHIER MIND, BREAST AND BODY.

BREAST-CARE *Journal*

Date: ___/___/___

○ Did self-breast exam this month? ○ Have any nipple discharge?

○ Have any new lumps or changes? ○ Did lymphatic breast massage?

○ Any visual size or shape changes? ○ Any pain or tenderness lately?

○ Any dimpling or redness? ○ Drank 6-8 glasses of water daily

○ Engaged in positive thinking ○ Have a clinical exam scheduled

○ Stretching /Yoga /Meditation ○ Ate nutrient-rich food?

○ Worked out 3x or more ○ Practice health gratitude

○ Annual Mammogram Scheduled

Add any additional health changes or concerns.

___

___

___

___

A LIFE OF GRATITUDE UNCLOCKS THE FULLNESS OF
A HEALTHIER MIND, BREAST AND BODY.

Breast Health Gratitude

Quietly practice a stress management of your choice & give yourself an affirmation of gratitude. Journal your experience.

A LIFE OF GRATITUDE UNCLOCKS THE FULLNESS OF
A HEALTHIER MIND, BREAST AND BODY.

BREAST-CARE *Journal*

Date: ___/___/___

- ◯ Did self-breast exam this month?
- ◯ Have any new lumps or changes?
- ◯ Any visual size or shape changes?
- ◯ Any dimpling or redness?
- ◯ Engaged in positive thinking
- ◯ Stretching /Yoga /Meditation
- ◯ Worked out 3x or more

- ◯ Have any nipple discharge?
- ◯ Did lymphatic breast massage?
- ◯ Any pain or tenderness lately?
- ◯ Drank 6-8 glasses of water daily
- ◯ Have a clinical exam scheduled
- ◯ Ate nutrient-rich food?
- ◯ Practice health gratitude

- ◯ Annual Mammogram Scheduled

Add any additional health changes or concerns.

___

___

___

___

A LIFE OF GRATITUDE UNCLOCKS THE FULLNESS OF
A HEALTHIER MIND, BREAST AND BODY.

Breast Health Gratitude

Quietly practice a stress management of your choice & give yourself an affirmation of gratitude. Journal your experience.

A LIFE OF GRATITUDE UNCLOCKS THE FULLNESS OF
A HEALTHIER MIND, BREAST AND BODY.

BREAST-CARE *Journal*

Date: ___/___/___

- ◯ Did self-breast exam this month?
- ◯ Have any new lumps or changes?
- ◯ Any visual size or shape changes?
- ◯ Any dimpling or redness?
- ◯ Engaged in positive thinking
- ◯ Stretching / Yoga / Meditation
- ◯ Worked out 3x or more

- ◯ Have any nipple discharge?
- ◯ Did lymphatic breast massage?
- ◯ Any pain or tenderness lately?
- ◯ Drank 6-8 glasses of water daily
- ◯ Have a clinical exam scheduled
- ◯ Ate nutrient-rich food?
- ◯ Practice health gratitude

- ◯ Annual Mammogram Scheduled

Add any additional health changes or concerns.

_____

_____

_____

_____

A LIFE OF GRATITUDE UNCLOCKS THE FULLNESS OF
A HEALTHIER MIND, BREAST AND BODY.

Breast Health Gratitude

Quietly practice a stress management of your choice & give yourself an affirmation of gratitude. Journal your experience.

A LIFE OF GRATITUDE UNCLOCKS THE FULLNESS OF
A HEALTHIER MIND, BREAST AND BODY.

www.ingramcontent.com/pod-product-compliance
Lightning Source LLC
Chambersburg PA
CBHW052030030426
42337CB00027B/4945